HEALING WITHIN:

The Complete Colon Health Guide

Written and Compiled by
Stanley Weinberger, C.M.T.

Copyright ©1988 by Stanley Weinberger
Colon Health Center
P.O. Box 1013
Larkspur, CA 94939

2nd Printing 1989

HEALING WITHIN: The Complete Colon Health Guide
can be purchased at most health food stores and bookstores.
For mail orders, see pages at the back of this book.

Book Design and Typesetting by Jana Janus, San Francisco, CA

ISBN 0-9616184-1-8

Printed in U.S.A.

Note to the Reader

HEALING WITHIN: The Complete Colon Health Guide does not claim to substitute for a physician's care, nor does it advocate specific solutions to individual problems. The physicians and experts providing the enclosed information have substantiated their claims as well as is possible considering that data on health and nutrition are subject to change as we learn more.

Before following the self-help advice given in this book, readers are earnestly urged to give careful consideration to the nature of their particular health problem and to consult a competent physician if they are in any doubt.

This book should not be regarded as a substitute for professional medical treatment. Every care has been taken to ensure accuracy of the content. Still, the author and publisher cannot accept legal responsibility for any problem arising out of the methods described in this book.

Dedication

Dedicated to Evelyn Wanek,
for all the many years of devoted service
you have given to colon therapy.
Bless you.

Table of Contents

CHAPTER 3
Colon Therapy: Pathway to Vibrant Health

CHAPTER 4
The Four- or Seven-Day Colon Cleansing Program

CHAPTER 5
Lactobacillus Acidophilus: The Well-kept Secret

CHAPTER 8
Metabolic Typing: The Commonsense Guide to Proper Nutrition

CHAPTER 9
Articles by Other Authors

CHAPTER 10
Quotes From America's Leading Experts on Colon Health

APPENDIX
Order Forms

List of Illustrations

About the Author
by Stanley Weinberger

Although I have been active in the health field for the past 18 years, my initial interest in health and finding ways to improve it was brought about by a severe decline in my own general state of health. I did not have a diagnosed disease, but still I was plagued with severe constipation, chronic back pain, excessive weight, constant fatigue, and irritability. I felt I was losing my zest for life and I was only in my mid-thirties.

After trying many different methods of treatment without showing improvement, I discovered colon therapy. Within six months and after approximately 30 treatments I had lost 70 pounds and began to regain my energy. The constipation improved and the nagging back pain all but disappeared. My outlook changed dramatically. I finally found a way to maintain and even improve my health.

Since that time, I have studied iridology (analyzing the iris of the eye for indications of bodily health and disease) with Dr. Bernard Jensen, and have studied metabolic nutrition with Dr. William Kelley and HEALTHEXCEL.

Currently, I am a Certified Metabolic Technician working with HEALTHEXCEL metabolic nutritional programs, iridology, and colon therapy. Eight years ago, I established the Colon Health Center in Marin County, ten miles north of San Francisco.

I want to acknowledge my editor, Beth Kuper. Without her this book would not have been possible. As an editor of three other books, she was a natural choice to edit *HEALING WITHIN: The Complete Colon Health Guide.*

Writing this book was inspired by my own health experiences and the desire to make information about the wonderful benefits of colon therapy and other valuable health practices more available to the general public.

Men occasionally stumble over the truth, but most pick themselves up and hurry off as if nothing had happened.

—Winston Churchill

Introduction

My purpose in writing this book is to familiarize you with a method of colon cleansing known as colonic irrigation, or colonics. This book also brings together the most current and relevant information from the works of some of the foremost authorities in the field of preventive medicine.

This new and revised edition of *HEALING WITHIN: The Complete Colon Health Guide* includes programs for parasite elimination and candida reduction, as well as an excellent inner-cleansing program and the very latest in nutritional support and metabolic-typing programs to assist you in strengthening your immune system.

Most of us recognize the importance of bringing our automobiles in for periodic tune-ups and maintenance. We all realize that unless we take proper care of the engine, carbon deposits and other buildup can reduce its efficiency and shorten its useful life. Yet we often go on for years, sometimes even for our whole lives, without giving a thought to the importance of inner cleansing of the most miraculous machine of all: our own bodies. But when you stop and think about it, nothing makes more sense.

A simple cleansing program is the first and most important positive step you can take to establish and maintain the highest possible level of health and vitality. Throughout your life, you are exposed to many varieties of air and water pollution, pesticides in food, and toxic chemicals in the environment. These, along with improper nutrition, stress, lack of exercise, and long-term use of prescription drugs can result in the loss of vitality, weakening of the immune system, sluggish eliminination and, eventually, illness. The buildup of toxins in the colon has an adverse effect on the whole body. This deterioration often takes place so slowly you may not even notice it; but nonetheless, it happens to everyone.

Colon cleansing is an effective, time-proven adjunct to any health or weight-loss program. This gentle method of cleansing and exercising the colon (large intestine) with warm water and herbs helps restore proper function and well-being to a very overworked and often toxic organ.

As you take more responsibility for your health habits, you learn to make decisions regarding your life-style that promote health, rather than hinder it. You contact a part of yourself that intuitively knows what is right for your emotional, physical, and spiritual health. You begin to release your fears.

You have the knowledge to heal yourself. All you have to do is begin to take charge of your body. Hopefully, this book will be an inspiration and guide to you in your quest for vibrant health.

Larkspur, California

January 1988

Colon therapy is not intended to be a cure-all, but is a valuable procedure for a wide variety of conditions of ill health. Intestinal malfunctions are precursors of many illnesses. The restoration of intestinal elimination, too often ignored, is an important preliminary course to the restoration of health. An inefficient colon is not always the cause of sickness, but it is believed to accentuate and prolong any and all diseased conditions of the human body.

—Dr. J.E.G. Waddington

CHAPTER 1

Your Colon Needs Attention!

Colon health is the most neglected and forgotten part of the body. Colon health emphasizes prevention rather than cure. It is the most important step in maintaining or regaining vital health.

—Norman W. Walker, D.Sc.

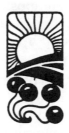

Colon Health

Your body is the house in which you live. By analogy, it is similar to the building in which you make your home. Your home needs, at the very least, periodic attention. Otherwise, the roof may leak, the plumbing may clog up, termites may drill through the floors and walls, and other innumerable signs of deterioration may make their appearance. Such is the case with your body. Every function and activity of your system, day and night, physical, mental, and emotional, is dependent upon the attention you give it.

The kind and quality of food you put into your body is of vital importance to every phase of your existence. Good nutrition regenerates the cells and tissues. It also enhances the processes by which waste matter, the undigested food, is eliminated from your body to prevent toxicity in the form of fermentation and putrefaction. This toxicity, if retained and allowed to accumulate in the body, prevents the possibility of attaining any degree of vibrant health.

The colon, a hollow tubelike organ also called the large intestine, extends from the cecum, where the small intestine empties the undigested food, and continues approximately five to five and a half feet down to the rectum.

The inner lining of the colon is equipped with sensitive nerves and glands. These glands aid the final stages of digestion and assimilation of food—especially minerals and water—and help to eliminate wastes from the system. Infrequent bowel movements or periods of constipation can result in only partial decomposition of these waste substances that encrust the colon. This further hinders elimination, causing a toxic buildup in the body.

Colon therapists and researchers in degenerative diseases have shown that much of the body weight can be just waste accumulated within the 60,000 miles of blood vessels, the lymphatic system, bone joints, and intra- and extracellular regions. The largest amount of waste is found in the impactions within the colon structures: up to 50 pounds of fecal waste can accumulate over the decades.

Some of this partially digested cooked food in the small intestine and colon passes into the bloodstream and is deposited as waste throughout the system. If these wastes are calories, they can show up as obesity; excess minerals show up as arthritis; excess protein is built into cancer; fat leads to high cholesterol; and sugar leads to diabetes.

In addition, the blood eliminates many of its wastes through the walls of the colon. When these wastes from the blood arrive at the inner walls of the colon, they are unable to pass through this area if it is crammed with hardened feces. So these wastes are reabsorbed and distributed throughout the body, poisoning the blood, weakening the immune system, and causing a variety of diseases.

Wastes, along with toxins resulting from the fermentation and putrefaction of undigested food, prevent muscular contractions (known as peristaltic waves) from sweeping the packed and hardened fecal matter along the digestive canal. The result of this condition is called intestinal stasis, or constipation.

When a person is constipated, the walls of the colon are packed with accumulated feces from many months or years of intestinal cramming. The colon might be compared to a water pipe that is partly obstructed by mineral deposits and corrosion. Thus, you can imagine how proper absorption of minerals into the bloodstream and elimination of feces would not occur in a congested and impacted colon. J.H. Tilden, M.D., said:

> *Without poisoning there can be no disease. In acute diseases we behold nature making her most profound effort to get rid of poison.*

Relief of this situation is not a simple matter of washing out loose material lying free inside the lower third of the colon. If this were the case, enemas would be sufficient for its removal.

Colonic irrigation, however, enables the impacted fecal matter to break down and be eliminated, along with particles of old mucous from the entire length of the colon. In some cases of cleansing, one or more forms of parasites, including tapeworms, may also be eliminated. Norman W. Walker, D.Sc., wrote:

> *The elimination of waste matter from the body should be meticulously taken care of by means of... colon irrigation whenever there is the slightest indication that the eliminative organs are becoming sluggish. In this eliminative washing out process, do not be misled into the thought that [colon cleansings] are not beneficial. Also disregard any claims that they cause loss of intestinal flora, as this is not true. No intestinal flora can exist or flourish when the fecal matter clogs up the glands in the colon that cause the flora to flourish.*

The very important intestinal bacteria (friendly flora) are damaged, weakened or destroyed by antibiotics, hormones, birth control pills, and steroids. By having colon cleansings and by orally taking a strong strain of acidophilus, you have the opportunity to rebuild the friendly bacterial level that may have been disrupted or destroyed by antibiotics, whether taken years ago or recently.

Unfortunately, no long-term side effect testing has been done on antibiotics, so the long-term side effects of these drugs are just beginning to emerge and be recognized. One of the side effects results in a yeast overgrowth (candida) in the colon that causes multiple health problems (see Chapter 6).

The Amazing Digestive System

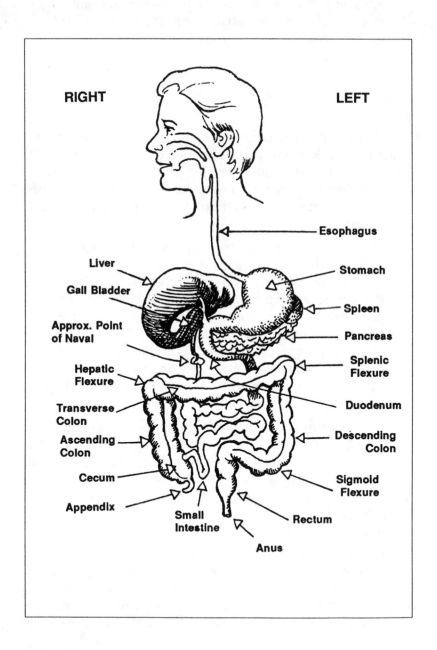

RIGHT

LEFT

Esophagus

Liver

Stomach

Gall Bladder

Spleen

Approx. Point
of Naval

Pancreas

Splenic
Flexure

Hepatic
Flexure

Duodenum

Transverse
Colon

Ascending
Colon

Descending
Colon

Cecum

Sigmoid
Flexure

Appendix

Small
Intestine

Rectum

Anus

The Length of the Human Digestive Tract as Compared to the Human Form

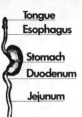

Tongue
Esophagus
Stomach
Duodenum
Jejunum

Small Intestine

Ileum
Cecum and Appendix
Colon
Rectum
Anus

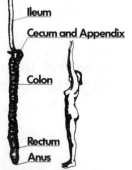

(Note that the length of the digestive tract is approximately six times longer than the human form.)

Each sack in your colon, found on the colon chart, is related to another part of your body. That is why colon cleansing helps different people in so many different ways.

—Norman W. Walker, D.Sc.

Colon Therapy Chart

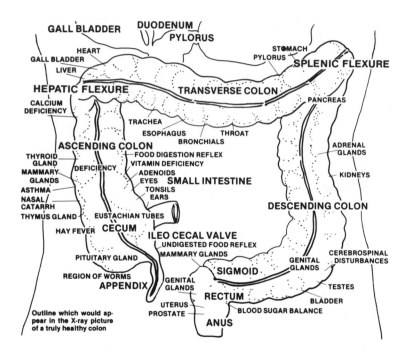

Colon therapy is recognized as an important step in maintaining or regaining health. The above chart illustrates how health and sickness have their roots in the colon. It is easy to see how an improper diet affects your colon and, in turn, inflicts pain or discomfort on the other parts of the body. Pocketing and buildup of fecal matter in various areas of the colon can affect those areas of the body indicated on the chart.

8

History of Colon Therapy

Despite treatment dating back to Biblical times, there still seems to be a great deal of ignorance about the healing benefits of colon therapy.

—Dr. J.E.G. Waddington

Colon therapy is a very ancient method of treatment and form of healing. Enemas were recorded as early as 1500 B.C. in the "Ebers Papyrus," an ancient Egyptian medical document. Hippocrates, Galen, and Pare also promoted the use of enema therapy. In these earlier times, people performed an enema in a lake or river using a hollow reed to allow water to flow into the rectum. Bernard Jensen, D.C., said:

In times past, knowledge of the bowel was more widespread and people were taught how to care for the bowel. Somehow, bowel wisdom got lost and it became something that no one wanted to talk about anymore.

Enemas were at one time a more common procedure than today. Before the departure of the Lewis and Clarke expedition, a physician instructed them in the appropriateness of using enemas in cases of fever and illness. Our grandparents and great-grandparents grew up with the use of enemas as a widely accepted procedure for reversing the onset of illness. The general public's awareness and practice of this valuable health tool has diminished greatly in the past 50 years. This is due to a deliberate attempt by the American Medical Association and the orthodox medical community to withhold vital information on the benefits of colon therapy, as well as many other preventive health practices.

With the development of sophisticated colonic irrigation machines and the increasing desire among many people to return to more natural methods of dealing with their health, colon therapy once again is experiencing a return to popularity. It is estimated that there may be as many as 2,000 therapists actively practicing colon therapy in the United States.

Do You Fit This Description?

Have you ever said, "I'm not constipated. I eliminate every day and I don't need a colon cleansing"?

Despite daily eliminations, many people are not aware that they may have a bowel problem. Very often, the complete length of the colon is impacted with old, hardened fecal matter, leaving only a narrow channel for smaller, softer feces to pass through. Failure to cleanse the colon is like having an entire garbage-collecting staff go on strike for months on end!

The colon is the sewage system of the body. If the wastes in the colon are allowed to build up, they will decay and absorb through the walls of the colon into the bloodstream. These toxins can poison the brain and nervous system so that you become depressed, irritable, weak, and listless; poison the lungs so that your breath is foul; poison the digestive system so that you are distressed and bloated; poison the blood so that your skin is sallow and unhealthy. In short, every organ is affected and you look and feel old, have stiff and painful joints, dull eyes, and sluggish thinking. Finally, you lose the joy of living. As Dr. Wager wrote about the Law of Disease:

Disease is a warning. It is a friend, not a foe, of mankind. It manifests itself in its various forms, from a slight cold to the more severe inflammations for the sole purpose of ridding the body of accumulated poisons.

Toxic Buildup

When people finally visit their doctor, they often have suffered for years from many of the following symptoms of toxic buildup and constipation:

- Fatigue and depression
- Gas-belching or flatulence
- Headaches

- Irritability, anxiety, nervousness
- Insomnia
- Nausea and abdominal discomfort
- Protruding, tender, or rigid abdomen
- Sagging posture
- Lack of interest in work or play
- Loss of memory or concentration
- Lack of sexual response
- Overweight, underweight, poor appetite, malnutrition
- Skin blemishes, sallow complexion, dark circles under the eyes
- Brittle hair and nails
- Bad breath, coated tongue, body odors
- Cold hands and feet
- Swelling of the legs
- Lower back pain
- Menstrual problems
- Blood pressure too high or too low
- Neuritis and neuralgia (aches and pains in different areas of the body)

Imbalances of the Colon

Structural, functional, and metabolic imbalances of the colon are manifested in various forms. The effects of autointoxication and constipation are shown in the most common abnormalities of the colon, such as adhesions, ballooning, colitis, diverticulitis, mucosal dysfunction, spastic bowel, strictures, and ulceration.

The following drawings illustrate the various abnormal shapes of the bowel in comparison to a normal bowel.

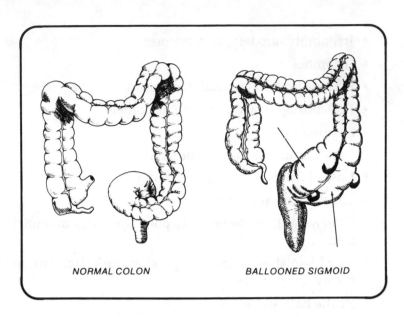

NORMAL COLON   BALLOONED SIGMOID

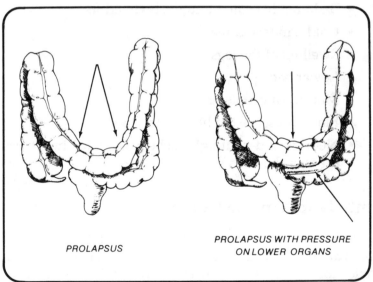

PROLAPSUS   PROLAPSUS WITH PRESSURE
ON LOWER ORGANS

Reprinted by permission of Bernard Jensen, D.C., Ph.D., from his book Tissue Cleansing Through Bowel Management, *1981.*

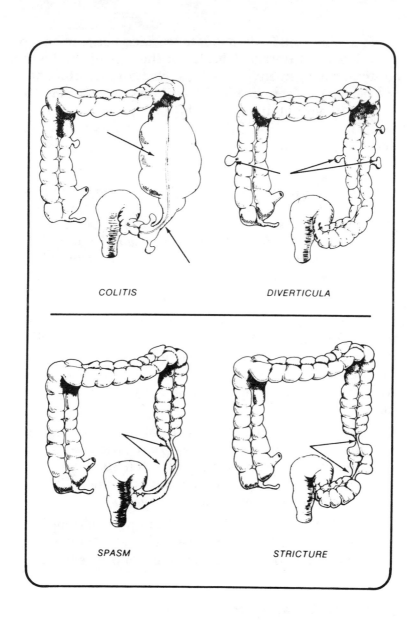

COLITIS

DIVERTICULA

SPASM

STRICTURE

Reprinted by permission of Bernard Jensen, D.C., Ph.D., from his book Tissue Cleansing Through Bowel Management, *1981.*

No doubt should exist about the relation between health of the intestinal tract and health in the rest of the body. Intestinal management probably is the most important factor a person can learn in a health-building routine. Some of the most important functions of life take place in the intestines. There, worn-out cells are eliminated and new cell structures are begun.

Attitudes that Promote Intestinal Inefficiency

By putting the bowel in the closet and making believe it doesn't exist, many people have gone down the path of improper living, treating the bowel indiscriminately and reaping the sad harvest in later years.

—Bernard Jensen, D.C., Ph.D.

Although incredible quantities of laxatives and stimulants are consumed by the general public each year, with or without professional advice or supervision (mostly without), the *causes* of intestinal problems are rarely examined. This unfortunate condition arises from the following viewpoints:

- A credulous public acceptance of many medical authorities who maintain that "Your bowels—like the universe—will get along very well if you leave them alone. They will adjust themselves to the body they inhabit and the kind of food you eat."

- A belief that constipation is an unimportant symptom, easily relieved by taking laxatives, bran, stimulants or other ineffective solutions to the real problem.

Causes of Constipation

- Too little liquid
- Too little bulk
- Too little exercise

- Emotional tension
- Mechanical problems, e.g., a prolapsed colon
- Poor choice of foods
- Improper combination of foods
- Temperature of foods too hot or too cold
- Weak muscle tone of the colon

Constipating Foods and Drinks

- Cheese
- Fried foods
- Candies and sugar products
- White flour
- Salt
- Salted snack foods (potato chips, etc.)
- Beef
- Canned, burned, fermented or processed foods
- Heavy, hardshelled or cellulose foods, such as tops of vegetables and legumes
- Pasteurized milk
- Wine with meals
- Carbonated drinks
- Coffee (has a drying effect on the colon)

If you are consuming these foods and drinks, your colon cannot possibly be healthy, even if you are having a bowel movement every day. Instead of furnishing nourishment to the nerves, muscle cells, and tissues of the walls of the colon, such substances can actually cause starvation of the colon. A starved colon may let a lot of fecal matter pass through it, but it is unable to carry on the last stages of digestion. Remember, cancer of the colon ranks next to heart disease as the most frequent cause of death in our country.

In order to be healthy, the body must be nourished properly. The colon produces a coat of mucous to protect itself from junk foods, pasteurized milk, preservatives, chemicals, and other pollutants. In time, this mucous coating can get as thick and hard as plastic. You can spend a fortune on vitamins, herbs, and organic foods, but the mucous coating prevents proper absorption of nutrients into your bloodstream. A colon cleansing does much to remove the excess mucous and to eliminate a toxic buildup from lining the walls of the colon. After a series of cleansings, you will experience a greater joy of living.

Attitudes that Promote Health

It is with love and self-respect that you establish for yourself a balanced life-style that promotes greater health. This includes cleansing the colon on a regular basis, exercise, fresh air, stress-release activities (meditation, massage, having fun), getting ample rest, drinking plenty of water, and eliminating drugs, processed foods, sugar, coffee, and other agents of disease from your diet.

Many people turn to colon cleansing when they find themselves in a state of disease or pain. Why not do so out of a desire to cleanse the body in order to achieve greater strength, mental awareness, and a sense of well-being? Knowing that you are in control of your body is the most important step toward realizing your health goals.

In his article "Gastrointestinal Therapy in Atrophic Arthritis," E. Goldfain, M.D., outlines his concepts for maintaining the digestive tract at its best.

A proper food supply: Adequate vitamins and minerals must be present, especially calcium, phosphorus and iron.

Good intestinal drainage: This is of paramount importance. If the bowel, especially the colon, is to function adequately, the amount and type of food that is ingested must be such as to avoid an excessive burden on the intestinal tract.

If the bulk of ingested food does not overload the lower digestive system, then the colon will automatically function more effectively. As Dr. Bernard Jensen tells us:

> *Bowel cleansing is an essential element in any lasting healing program. The toxic waste must be removed as quickly as possible to halt this downward spiral of failing health.*

Colon Reflex Chart

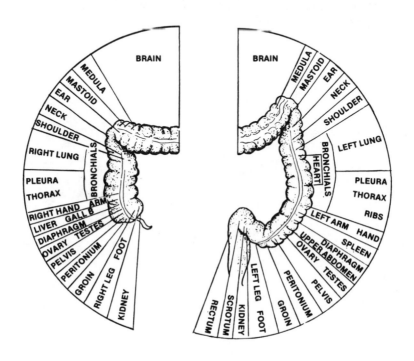

The colon produces reflex conditions in various organs in the body. In the above chart, the organ opposite the particular part of the bowel shows the part of the body affected directly by the colon. Symptoms in various parts of the body are relieved and many times eliminated when the intestinal flora have been changed. No matter what conditions we have in the body, they are affected by the bowel whether it is good or bad.

Reprinted from Science & Practice of Iridology, by Bernard Jensen, D.C., N.D., Escondido, CA, 1952.

CHAPTER 2

Suggestions to Improve Bowel Function

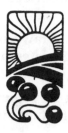

Suggestions to Improve Bowel Function

In addition to colon cleansing, you can improve your bowel function and feeling of well-being by consuming the proper foods and liquids, combining and cooking foods correctly, and exercising and meditating regularly.

- At least 50 percent of the foods you eat should be "live"— fresh, raw, and unprocessed (preferably organic). Dead foods cannot build strong bodies. Eat foods in season.

- Have your main meal as early in the day as possible. Eat two thirds of your daily intake before mid-afternoon. Do not go to sleep at night on a full stomach.

- Chew your food well; at least 10 to 20 chews for each mouthful.

- Do not eat if ill or emotionally upset; do not overeat.

- Eat the following daily: six vegetables, two fruits, one starch, and one protein. Vary these foods from meal to meal and from day to day.

- Eat at least one full serving of a whole grain daily, such as millet, brown rice or yellow cornmeal.

- Eat at least two full servings of raw or cooked vegetables daily, including one serving of such vegetables as cabbage, brussel sprouts or sauerkraut.

- Eat foods (greens) containing potassium and sodium.
- Eat two ounces of fresh sprouts daily: bean, mung, fenugreek, pea.
- Eat at least one pound of raw fruit daily: apples, bananas, papaya, pineapple, figs, dates, prunes. Always soak dried fruit overnight in apple juice and eat for breakfast.
- Eat at least one pint of yogurt daily, preferably goat yogurt. Also add kefir (not sweetened with sugar) to your diet.
- Eat one ounce of unfiltered honey daily with yogurt or tea.
- Eat lots of fibrous foods.

Liquids to Improve Bowel Function

- Drink sufficient liquids (water, juices, herbal teas): one-half ounce daily for each pound of body weight. For example, if you weigh 128 pounds, you should drink 64 ounces (8 cups) of liquids daily.
- Do not drink liquids with meals. Take liquids between meals using distilled or filtered water, unsweetened juices, herbal teas or grain beverages.
- Drink eight ounces of goat milk daily. Warm the milk and sip it slowly.

Food Combining and Amounts

- Select 70 percent of your daily food intake from alkaline-forming foods; 30 percent from acid-forming foods.
- It's easier on your digestive system if you do not eat fruits and vegetables at the same meal. Have fruit for breakfast and a mid-afternoon snack.
- Starch and protein do not combine well. Have one at lunch, the other at dinner. It's best to eat protein in the morning and at noon, rather than in the evening.

Alkaline-Forming Foods

Fruit juices, goat's milk, vegetable juices, potatoes, fruits, vegetables, raw honey, sprouting seeds.

Acid-Forming Foods

Meat, fish, fowl, cheese, eggs, rice, bread, cereal, peanuts, nuts, sugar (avoid), citrus juices.

Foods to Avoid or Replace

- Avoid nuts or peanut butter.

- Avoid very hot or very cold food or liquids.

- Eliminate fried foods of all kinds; instead, bake, broil or steam your foods.

- Avoid pork and pork products (lunch meats, hot dogs, ham, bacon, etc.). Many parasites in pork are heat resistant.

- If you are a red-meat eater, reduce your daily intake to two ounces or less. Replace red meat with fish or fowl whenever possible. Always purchase poultry, beef, and other animal products that haven't been fed antibiotics and growth hormones. These additives destroy the vital intestinal flora, are carcinogenic, and damage bowel function. Many health food stores now carry range-fed poultry. The cost is slightly higher but well worth the price difference.

- Replace table salt (NaCl) with Dr. Jensen's Seasoning Powder or Bio-Salt. If you must use salt, use sea salt (naturally evaporated) rather than iodized salt.

Cooking Suggestions

- Do not use aluminum or Teflon™ cookware because tiny particles of metal or coatings chip off and leach into the food. Also, the oxidation process of cooking in aluminum is harmful to foods. Use stainless steel whenever possible.
- Do not wrap food in aluminum foil unless the food is first wrapped in plastic.
- Cook with low heat; cook with little water and cover the pan. Cook vegetables as little as possible. Crock pots will retain a majority of nutrients in food.
- Do not fry foods; instead, bake, broil or steam them.

Bowel Function

- Take all laxatives out of your medicine cabinet and throw them away.
- The most beneficial time of day for bowel elimination is early in the morning, either before or soon after breakfast.
- Make a habit to try to have a bowel movement first thing in the morning, whether you receive the call or not. Allow at least 15 minutes; do not strain. Remember, weak bowels take more time to function. Breathing deeply and bending the head toward the knees while in the sitting or squatting position can help.
- Take pleasure and pride in your bowel health.

Exercise and Meditation

- Develop some form of deep-breathing and meditation exercises.
- Express your feelings more—loosen up! Constipation can be associated with the refusal to release old ideas. Try this affirmation each day: "I release the past. I generously allow life to flow through me."
- Do plenty of exercise daily: walking, running, jumping, bending, stretching, yoga, self-massage, and slant-board exercises.

Slant-Board Exercises
*For Prolapsed Colon and Regenerating
the Vital Nerve Centers of the Brain*

Reprinted by permission of Bernard Jensen, D.C., Ph.D.,
from his book *Tissue Cleansing Through
Bowel Management*, 1981.

Slant-board exercises are absolutely necessary to regaining perfect health. These exercises are a vital means to increase blood flow to the brain, tone the muscles, and improve circulation to all areas of the body.

When there is a lack of tone in the muscles of the colon, you can expect prolapsus (a dropping) of the abdominal organs. If the body lacks tone, the heart cannot circulate blood properly. Likewise, arteries and veins cannot contract to help move the blood against gravity into the brain tissues.

Slant-board exercises are practically the same as any other lying-down exercises and are especially good in cases of inflammations and congestions above the neck. This includes sinus trouble, failing eyesight, hair loss, head eczema, ear conditions, and similar problems. Slant-board exercises have helped in cases of heart trouble, fatigue, dizziness, poor memory, and paralysis.

There are some people who have tried nearly everything to get well and who still find all organs working under par. Many people do not realize that all the quickening force for every organ of the body comes from the brain. The heart gets its start from the brain and continues its everlasting pumping because of it. People whose occupations require them to sit or stand continually are unable to get the blood into the brain tissues because the tired organs cannot force the blood uphill. If the brain tissues are denied good blood in the proper amount, in time every organ in the body will suffer.

There are some cases where the slant board is contraindicated. It is usually best to get professional advice, for some people have had unhappy experiences because they started with too strenuous a program. If you haven't done much exercising of the abdominal muscles, it is well to take these exercises slowly and gradually increase them as you get stronger.

Do not use the board in cases of high blood pressure, hemorrhages, some tubercular conditions, cancer in the pelvic cavity, appendicitis, ulcers of the stomach or intestines, or pregnancy, unless under the care of a physician.

Directions for Using the Slant Board

Rest the head end of the board on the floor and put the foot end at chair height for all exercises. If you become dizzy at first, don't raise the foot end of the board quite so high to begin with.

In the beginning, do slant-board exercises only five minutes a day; more than that is too much. As you become more accustomed to the exercises, gradually increase time spent on the board.

The following numbered exercises correspond to the illustrations.

1. Lie full length, allowing gravity to help the abdominal organs into their position. For best results, lie on the board at least 10 minutes, preferably at mid-afternoon and again just before going to bed. After retiring, lift the buttocks up to allow the organs to return to their normal position.

2. While lying flat on your back, stretch the abdomen by putting arms above head. Bring arms above head 10 to 15 times; this stretches the abdominal muscles and pulls the abdomen down toward the shoulders.

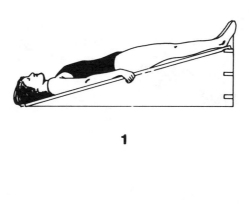

1

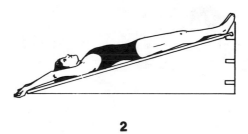

2

3. Bring abdominal organs toward shoulders while holding your breath. Move the organs back and forth by drawing them upward, contracting abdominal muscles, and then allowing them to go back to a relaxed position. Do this 10 to 15 times.

4. Pat abdomen vigorously with open hands. Lean to one side, then to the other, patting the stretched side. Pat 10 to 15 times each side.

Bring the body to sitting position, using the abdominal muscles. Return to lying position. Do this three to four times, if possible. Do only if your doctor orders.

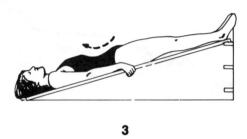

3

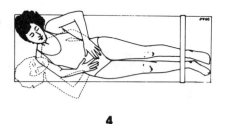

4

Hold on to the sides of the board while doing the following exercises.

5. Bend knees and legs at hips. While in this position (a) turn head from side to side five or six times, and (b) lift head slightly and rotate in circles three or four times.

6. Lift legs to vertical position, rotate outward in circles eight or ten times. Increase to 25 times after a week or two of exercising.

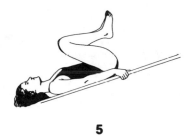

5

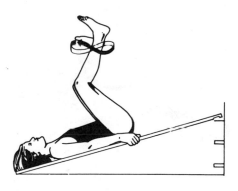

6

7. Bring legs straight up to a vertical position and lower them to the board slowly. Repeat three or four times.

8. Bicycle legs in air 15 to 25 times.

   Relax and rest, letting blood circulate in the head for 10 minutes.

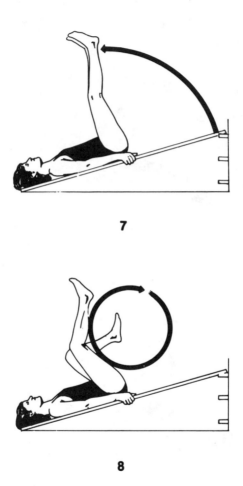

7

8

Reprinted by permission of Bernard Jensen, D.C., Ph.D., from his book Tissue Cleansing Through Bowel Management, *1981.*

The Ileocecal Valve Syndrome

by Dr. David G. Williams

Every so often I run into a technique or method of helping people that is so dramatic and simple to use that I wish the whole world could be aware of it. Techniques involving the ileocecal valve (ill-lee-o-see-cal) are a good example of this.

Wouldn't it be nice to know something to do when you or your family had a sudden case of diarrhea or constipation? Or wouldn't it be nice to stop those so-called flu-type symptoms that so often hit with absolutely no warning? When the ileocecal valve isn't working right, it can cause these symptoms and many more. Just look at the list of things that it can cause:

shoulder pain	light-headedness
nausea	ringing in the ear
dizziness	lower back pain for no reason
chest pains	recurrent sinus infections
heart fluttering	headaches and fever
bursitislike pain in the shoulders and hip joints	

What and Where Is This Valve?

The ileocecal valve is located between the small and large intestine. Basically, it is located in the same area as the appendix and many times what is thought to be an appendix problem is instead a problem with the valve. This little valve has two very important jobs to do. First, it serves as a block that prevents the toxic contents of the large intestine from backing up into the small intestine. Second, it keeps the food products in the small intestine from passing into the large intestine before the digestive processes have been completed.

The valve can at times become either stuck shut or stuck open. When stuck shut, the ileocecal valve can cause constipation, and when stuck open, diarrhea will be the problem.

When the Valve Sticks Shut

Food becomes toxic after staying in the body too long. It should move on through the large intestine and then be expelled by the body. Sometimes, if the valve sticks shut, the feces or toxic waste material will have to stay in the small intestine and will be unable to move any further. Naturally, since the small intestine's job is to absorb, it keeps right on working and absorbing all of the waste products and garbage into the body! Also, with the valve shut and the food backing up, you become constipated.

When the Valve Sticks Open

By sticking open, the ileocecal valve not only allows food to move through you at a rapid rate (to say the least), but it also lets the waste products in the large intestine back up into the small intestine and again be reabsorbed into the system!

It doesn't take a genius to realize that the valve can cause a world of problems, but better yet, it doesn't take a genius to do some easy things to help stabilize the valve.

Why Me?

There are several reasons why the valve doesn't always work right, but I'll only mention a few of the more common ones here. Sometimes spicy or roughage-type foods will irritate the valve and cause it to stick shut or open. Another factor that greatly influences the valve is stress or emotional trauma. Almost everyone is exposed to these factors, but some of us are more sensitive than others. I personally find that those who have had their appendix removed seem to have more problems. Some researchers believe that the appendix, which is located right next to the valve, acts like "an overflow bag for toxins" and holds these until the body can work them slowly and not interrupt the workings of the ileocecal valve.

Open Ileocecal Valve, What to Do

When the valve is open (diarrhea, loose stools, and symptoms like those mentioned earlier), there are some temporary things that can be done first. The valve is located on the right side, about halfway between the belly button and the hip bone. Many times you can get relief in one of two ways.

First, you can sometimes hold the valve shut for several minutes. This is done by placing your hand over the valve and while pushing in, pull up toward the left shoulder.

The second way is to place a cold pack made of cold water or ice over the valve for about 15 to 20 minutes. This process can be repeated if necessary.

Stopping the Flu Dead in Its Tracks

Except for the two things to do for diarrhea and an open ileocecal valve (which I also find works quite well for travelers in Mexico who are suffering from the famous so-called *tourista* or Montezuma's revenge), there are several things that need to be done for both the open and the closed valve.

When I find this problem with one of my patients or if I have a patient suffering from either diarrhea or constipation, I instruct the patient as follows:

1. First, the toxic food products that are either backing up or that are blocked up in the intestines need to be detoxified and the best method to do this is to use either garlic or chlorophyll. I find that chlorophyll works best and is easy to obtain at any health food store. Initially, either two capsules or tablets or one half teaspoon of chlorophyll liquid should be taken every two hours for about six to eight hours and the same amount with each meal for the next three to four days.

2. Next, the diet should be modified to eliminate spicy foods for a week or so. If the problem is diarrhea, it is also helpful to eliminate all roughage-type food for a short

33

period of time. If the ileocecal valve is closed and constipation is a problem, then increase the roughage.

3. Alcohol, cocoa, chocolate, and caffeine products should be eliminated.

4. With a closed valve (constipation), add calcium and vitamin D to the diet.

5. With an open valve (diarrhea), add to the diet a product called lactic acid yeast, which can be obtained at any health food store. This product alone can sometimes stop even the most stubborn cases of chronic diarrhea.

6. MOST IMPORTANT OF ALL, BY RUBBING ON THE FOLLOWING "REFLEX" POINTS FOR BOTH THE OPEN AND THE CLOSED ILEOCECAL VALVE, YOU CAN RELIEVE THE PROBLEM ALMOST INSTANTLY!

The areas illustrated in the diagram on page 35 should be massaged with firm pressure for about 10 to 20 seconds each (it is not beneficial to rub the points any longer than that; in fact, it may negate the effect).

Most of the points will be extremely sore if the problem is long standing. Ask a cooperative friend to work out the points, or use a vibrator.

The next time you first start to get the flulike symptoms of achiness, fatigue or sore throat, or the next time you or a member of your family start to have problems with either constipation or diarrhea, try rubbing on these reflex points. You might be surprised to find that your problem may leave in a matter of minutes instead of weeks!

Reprinted from Alternatives, *Vol. 1, No. 3, a monthly health newsletter written by Dr. David G. Williams, published by Mountain Home Publishing, P.O. Box 829, Ingram, TX 78025. Subscription price $39 per year.*

Ileocecal Valve Reflex Points

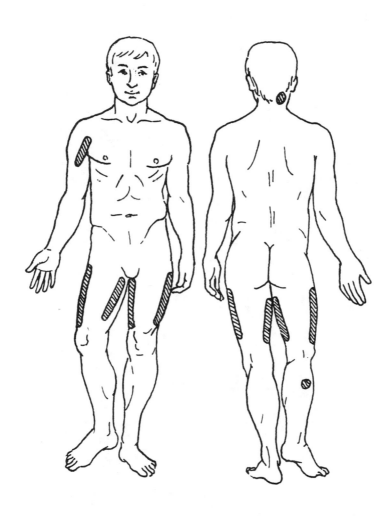

The areas illustrated should be massaged with firm pressure for about *10 to 20 seconds* each (it is not beneficial to rub the points any longer than that; in fact, it may negate the effect).

CHAPTER 3

Colon Therapy: Pathway to Vibrant Health

Although colon health emphasizes prevention, many people have found relief from constipation, fatigue, poor eyesight, hearing loss, asthma, prostate trouble, colds, allergies, nagging backache, respiratory disorders, digestive problems, gas, abdominal pain, colitis, indigestion, overweight, nutritional deficiencies, hypoglycemia, depression, anxiety, tenseness, and numerous other ailments.

—Norman W. Walker, D.Sc.

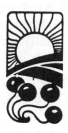

Benefits of Colon Therapy

Colon therapy is a restorative, relaxing experience that is both pleasant and effective. Most people report relief of problems after the very first treatment. Vitality and energy levels are restored. Colon therapy has an antiseptic and solvent action on the intestines, whereby putrefactive material, impacted fecal matter, excess mucous, and even pus and infected tissue are removed from the colon. This leaves a cleaner, healthier colon, which means a healthier body.

Colon therapy increases the water level and diuretic action of the body. Water is absorbed into the body, which increases the volume of the blood. Circulation is thereby increased, resulting in greater bathing of the individual cells, thus diluting toxins and flushing them out; relieving uremia and toxemia; and increasing elimination both through kidneys and skin as well as the bowel. All this generally assists the cardiovascular and circulatory systems' efficiency.

During a colon cleansing, both warm and cool water may be used. The warm water supplies heat to the body. The cleansing action along with the warm temperature is excellent for relieving colds and flu. Probably the greatest benefit of bathing the colon in warm water is relief from tension and irritability. X-rays following treatment demonstrate that spastic colons are more relaxed and relieved of muscle spasms as well as the swelling, irritation, and inflammation of tissues that accompany this problem.

On the other hand, the effects of cool water can also be beneficial. Any time there is a fever, cool water will aid in reducing it. Swollen tissues can be alleviated and a loose or elongated colon can also be improved. A colon lacking tone, accompanied by gas and constipation, will benefit greatly by the stimulation of the cleansing, which induces peristalsis.*

Many colon X-rays show that pressure of constipation is exerted in the liver area, resulting in irritation to both liver and gall bladder, as well as to the common bile duct. This delays and obstructs the normal draining of these organs— a condition that is often alleviated through colon therapy.

In some cases, pain in the heart area is also relieved. X-rays demonstrate that parts of the colon can be very high in the upper left quadrant causing irritation to the heart. Rapid heartbeat, hypertension, and various chest pains may all be alleviated by proper intestinal cleansing.

Many overweight patients have eliminated as much as 10 to 25 pounds by having their intestinal tract cleansed. Constipation is responsible for the accumulation of large amounts of fecal matter in that area as well as allowing the body wastes to build up at the cellular level. Proper colon cleansing aids greatly in eliminating unwanted and unsightly excess pounds—not to mention that dull, irritable feeling that is so prevalent. Unfortunately, weight gain comes upon people so gradually that they often don't realize what changes occur from year to year.

Various other results are often seen. Some patients report they have never been able to perspire until receiving colon therapy. Because of the removal of toxic wastes, the skin becomes strong and healthy and people look years younger. Memory is often improved. A feeling of well-being hastens the removal of bowel contents (mucous, gas, parasites, undigested food particles, glandular and cellular debris, plus bacterial toxins).

---

*The wavelike muscular contractions and dilations of the colon that move the contents forward.

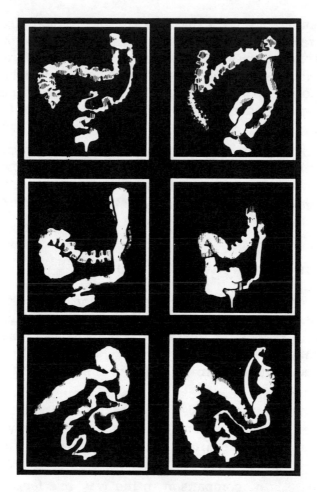

The above six pictures of prolapsed, distorted, twisted, sickly looking colons are exact reproductions of X-ray negatives of the colons of apparently healthy, civilized people whose illusions about their physical condition were exploded when they saw this conclusive evidence.

Civilized life means an artifical life; civilized people, living in a civilized manner and eating civilized foods, cannot, in the very nature of things, have a truly **healthy colon**.

Health and sickness both have their roots in the **colon**.

—Dr. Norman W. Walker, D.Sc.

41

Gentle abdominal massage during a colon cleansing helps release fecal impactions, moving the water around to help break up the solidified crust on the inner surface of the colon. It also stimulates peristalsis and helps return the colon to its normal shape, thus removing pressure on other organs (liver, gall bladder, stomach, heart, etc.). Dr. Bernard Jensen wrote:

> *Every person who desires the higher things in life must be aware of proper bowel management, what it is, how it works, and what is required. In so doing, you will discover many secrets of life, develop a positive attitude toward yourself, and become the master of body function.*

Colon Therapy with Oxygen

In recent years, a new approach to colon therapy has been introduced. By mixing medically pure oxygen with the water used to flush the colon, therapists have achieved miraculous results. Those patients who previously had colon cleansings report many differences in the results.

Colon therapy with oxygen has a definite calming effect on the nervous system. Nervousness and irritability are both lessened. A person not only becomes easier to live with, but feels so much better from both improved nerve functions and having eliminated toxins that irritate the nerves.

There is no comparison in the way one feels after a cleansing with the new procedure with oxygen. In fact, it is reported that the small blood vessels lining the colon instantly absorb oxygen—normalizing not only the lower bowel, but also the entire body. Some authorities state that, liter per liter, more oxygen is absorbed through colon cleansing than through the lungs. This not only helps to heal the affected tissues in the colon, but also allows the oxygen to pass quickly into the bloodstream and bathe all the cells in the body.

Oxygen aids in the healing of sores and wounds. In many cases, acidophilus or lactobacilli (the friendly bacteria) have been destroyed by improper eating habits, constipation, diarrhea, parasites, an infected colon, and antibotics. Affected areas in the colon, resulting in irritation, infection, colitis, ulceration, and diverticulosis are bathed with a continuous supply of their life-supporting element, oxygen, which hastens healing in the colon as well as other parts of the body.

Colon therapy with oxygen has an anthelmintic action; that is, parasites are removed. Many patients are found to have some form of parasites, the most common being tapeworm. Various other types found are hookworms, pinworms, roundworms, whipworms, and many other exotic forms. Sources of tapeworms are usually beef, pork or fish. Many vegetarians also are infected with various parasites by eating vegetables or fruit infested with parasite eggs. Dr. Norman Walker said:

> *Experience has taught me that no health and healing procedures can be as successful as those which have a series of colon irrigations as the prelude to any health treatment. This makes sense because just so long as there is material in the colon which may be conducive to the generation of poisons in the colon and to the diffusion of such poisons throughout the system, no healing can take place which is not the precursor of a chain reaction of ailments at a future date.*

Colon-Cleansing Procedure

A colon cleansing is a gentle, warm-water washing of the colon (large intestine) combined with some external massage. Also known as intestinal hydrotherapy or colonic irrigation, it is completely safe, beneficial, and nontoxic.

The procedure lasts approximately 45 minutes and is performed by a colon therapist using a colon irrigation machine that regulates the water pressure, temperature, and water volume. A five-inch speculum attached to a hose (both disposable) is inserted into the anus, allowing the water to flow in under gentle pressure to cleanse the entire length of the colon. The water dislodges toxic wastes in the colon, which are then flushed out through the waste hose. During a cleansing, a series of water-fills and releases also helps to stimulate the expansion and contraction of the muscular walls of the colon. This, combined with a changing of the water temperature from warm to cool, exercises the colon and promotes the restoration of proper peristaltic action.

During the cleansing, most people find that they can relax completely. After the cleansing is completed, acidophilus can be taken to increase the level of beneficial flora present in the intestinal tract.

Note: Since nearly all tap water contains chemicals as well as other undesirable substances, it is most important that the water used in a colon cleansing be purified by some form of filtration system.

Most up-to-date colonic machines are equipped with disposable hoses and speculums to insure cleanliness. You should insist on disposable accessories that are used only once and then thrown away.

Commonly Asked Questions About Colon Therapy

Q: Are colon cleansings completely safe?

A: Yes. In fact, with the new Toxygen equipment (an oxygen-equipped colon cleansing machine), treatments are much safer than the common enema.

Q: How does a colon cleansing compare to an enema?

A: An enema only bathes the lower part of the colon, whereas a colon cleansing bathes the entire length of the colon, approximately five to five and a half feet. A colon cleansing is many more times effective, according to learned centenarian Dr. Norman Walker, who said, "One colonic is equivalent to 30 enemas."

Q: Do treatments hurt?

A: No. In fact, with the advanced equipment now available, treatments are refreshing and relaxing.

Q: How much of the intestines are actually cleansed during a colon cleansing?

A: During a treatment we are actually able to bathe the full length of the colon, but we are not able to cleanse the small intestine. The buildup in the small intestine is cleared with the help of the Intestinal Cleanser and other nutritional aids taken orally during a series of cleansings.

Q: Should I see my doctor before having a colon cleansing?

A: If there is something organically or internally wrong, it's always a good idea to consult your doctor. However, since colon cleansings professionally administered with the new Toxygen equipment are safer than home enemas, a medical examination is not required except for those who are ill.

Q: How long does a treatment take?

A: Between 35 and 45 minutes, but you should plan for an hour stay.

Q: Does having a menstrual period at the time of the cleanse have any effect on the success of the treatment?

A: No, in fact it's usually a good time to receive a treatment, since your body is already cleansing. Your menstrual flow will not interfere with the success of the treatment. Flushing the colon will also reduce abdominal pressure associated with menstrual cycles.

Q: What should I do to prepare for a colon cleansing?

A: Refrain from eating before the cleansing, be as relaxed as possible, and maintain a positive, cheerful attitude. Do not drink carbonated beverages.

Q: Is there any possibility of bacterial or viral contamination from prior use of the colonic machine?

A: That's a very timely question. The latest colonic machines now use presterilized disposable hoses and speculums. Since these accessories are only used once and then thrown away, there is no danger of contamination.

Q Will I experience any intestinal discomfort or fatigue after the cleansing?

A: Not usually, but since the cleansing will stir up a lot of old debris and toxins, you might experience some nausea or fatigue. I recommend resting and applying a warm heating pad to the abdomen if any discomfort occurs. A mild vegetable broth or peppermint tea is usually soothing at this time. Any discomfort will usually pass within 24 hours.

Q: Do I need to use acidophilus after a colon cleansing because the treatment washes out flora from the colon?

A: I recommend using acidophilus, but not because the treatment has washed out the flora. Colon cleansings don't wash out flora. I urge the use of acidophilus because it is an opportunity to improve the bacterial balance in the colon. I recommend taking acidophilus capsules during a cleansing program and continuing for at least 60 days afterward. (See Chapter 5 for more information on acidophilus.)

Q: Can I work after a colon cleansing?

A: Certainly. Colon cleansing should not interfere with your scheduled day.

CHAPTER 4

The Four- or Seven-Day Colon Cleansing Program

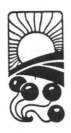

Four- or Seven-Day
Colon Cleansing Program

Colon cleansing treatments are the central focus of this program, since so much toxic buildup accumulates in the colon. The colon cleansing treatments remove much of the old waste material and mucous buildup. These treatments will help cleanse your elimination organs: the skin, kidneys, lungs, liver, bowel, and lymphatic system. The cleansing program is not represented as a cure for any disease or ailment. It is simply a method of cleansing the body to help create a healthier YOU.

The cleanse is not to be considered a weight-loss program, but it is not unusual to lose five to seven pounds during the course of the four to seven days. Since the cleansing process helps improve digestion, assimilation, and elimination, additional weight loss may occur even when you return to solid foods.

Please observe as closely as possible all instructions and the suggested schedule on the following pages. Each product and procedure has its purpose and should produce wonderful results.

Note: I do not recommend that you attempt this program without some form of colon cleansing. Enemas are helpful, but colonics work best and are more thorough.

The program will seldom conflict with any other therapy or treatment, but if you are presently under a doctor's care, it is best to discuss this program with your physician and seek his or her counsel and support. If your doctor is interested in preventive health care, he or she will understand that a clean body will be more responsive to any therapeutic measures that you may need.

The program is not intended to replace qualified medical care. I recommend that the seriously ill and the elderly go easy with this program, seeking the advice of their doctor in modifying any of these procedures to conform to individual specific needs and limitations.

Instructions

The following is a step-by-step instruction guide for the Four- or Seven-Day Colon Cleansing Program.

If you are doing the Four-Day Cleansing Program, you should begin all products on Day 1. You should receive colon cleansings on Days 2, 3, and 4 of the program.

If you are doing the Seven-Day Cleansing Program, you should begin all products on Day 1. You should receive colon cleansings on Days 2, 3, 5, and 7 of the program.

- Eat nothing else during the cleansing program other than what is specified in these instructions.
- Discontinue all vitamin and mineral supplements during the cleansing program.
- Drink distilled, bottled or filtered water (six to eight glasses daily), herbal teas, Bernard Jensen's broth, and diluted fresh vegetable and fruit juices. Lots of liquids are essential for best results. Avoid orange, pineapple, and grapefruit juices at this time, due to their high acid content. Do not drink canned, artificially flavored or carbonated beverages during the cleansing program.
- Exercise moderately every day. The best exercise is a brisk walk, but always use good judgment and don't push yourself if you're fatigued.

- Avoid TV and movies at this time. Body cleansings are quiet times and are excellent opportunities to catch up on reading or listening to soothing music.
- Get a good night's rest, at least eight hours of sleep.
- Begin all products and procedures on the morning of Day 1. Your first colon cleansing will be on Day 2.

Products and Procedures

Apple Cider Vinegar Drink

Apple cider vinegar contains lots of potassium and is helpful in relieving mucous from the body. It is important to drink it immediately after you take the Intestinal Cleansing caplets.

Instructions: Mix one tablespoon of apple cider vinegar with eight ounces of hot water. You may add a teaspoon of maple syrup if desired. Stir and drink at a moderate temperature. Follow it with an eight ounce glass of water.

Bernard Jensen's Broth

This broth is loaded with vitamins and minerals. You will find it very satisfying during the cleansing, especially at dinner time. However, you can drink it as often as you wish. After your cleansing, try it as a substitute seasoning for salt and pepper. It is delicious on vegetables, salads, meat, or any cooked foods (do not use on fruit).

Instructions: Mix one teaspoon of Bernard Jensen's Broth with eight ounces of hot water, stir, and drink.

Bilax Tablets

Bilax is a mild herbal stool softener that acts only on the colon. The Bilax tablets will help reduce mucous as well as soften stools for more effective results during your colon cleansings.

Instructions: Take two Bilax tablets at bedtime on evenings before your colon cleansings.

If you are on the Four-Day Cleansing Program, take two Bilax tablets on the evenings of Days 1, 2, and 3.

If you are on the Seven-Day Cleansing Program, take two Bilax tablets on the evenings of Days 1, 2, 4, and 6.

Discontinue use of Bilax after the cleansing program.

Castor Oil Packs for the Immune System

Edgar Cayce, an acclaimed health practitioner, recommended castor oil packs in thousands of his psychic health readings. Although there has never been an extensive study of the medicinal effects of castor oil packs, it has been found that applying this oil as a heat pack on the abdomen has a profound relaxing and regenerative effect on the whole body. Beneficial results can be seen in the lymphatic system. Many of Cayce's recorded case histories indicate marvelous results. Cayce also recommended these packs be applied on nights before colon cleansings to relax and tone the colon.

Instructions: Gather together several large plastic garbage bags, several towels, a heating pad, a bowl, and the castor oil. Pour four ounces of castor oil into the bowl and soak the flannel cloth in the oil. Spread a plastic garbage bag on your bed with a towel on top of it and lie down on the towel.

Apply the cloth evenly to the general region of your abdomen. Next, put another large garbage bag over the cloth and tuck the bag under you. Place a towel over the plastic and apply the heating pad. Leave on for one to one and a half hours on low heat.

When this is completed, place the flannel cloth in a plastic bag and store it in the refrigerator. Apply the castor oil pack each evening before the day of the colon cleansing.

If you are on the Four-Day Cleansing Program, apply the castor oil pack on the evenings of Days 1, 2, and 3.

If you are on the Seven-Day Cleansing Program, apply the castor oil pack on the evenings of Days 1, 2, 4, and 6.

DDS-1 Acidophilus Culture

DDS-1 Acidophilus culture is one of just a few brands of acidophilus that is acid resistant and can survive the long journey through the digestive tract to the colon. DDS-1 delivers one billion friendly bacteria in each capsule. These bacteria will colonize and reestablish the much needed friendly flora that may be absent due to past antibiotic use. DDS-1 helps improve bowel movements and also has an excellent cleansing effect on the liver. Acidophilus is also known to reduce blood cholesterol levels.

DDS-1 should be taken with water only, the first thing in the morning and at bedtime. DDS-1 should not be taken with food or other liquids because these substances would stimulate the natural stomach acids, which would weaken the ability of DDS-1 to recolonize in the colon.

Instructions: Take two DDS-1 Acidophilus capsules first thing in the morning and again at bedtime, with water only. Be sure to refrigerate the DDS-1 Acidophilus capsules to keep the bacteria stable.

Dry Skin Brushing

Dry skin brushing is the finest method I know to cleanse the skin. The skin should eliminate up to two pounds of wastes daily; skin brushing helps remove uric acid crystals, mucous, and other acids from the body. When the skin retains these waste materials, many of them are reabsorbed into the bloodstream. Brushing each day will keep your skin looking good and will reduce toxic buildup throughout your body.

You may find at first that the bristles feel very scratchy; this is normal. These are vegetable bristles and are not harmful to your skin. Just brush lightly until you become used to the sensation. After a few days, you will find that the brushing has stimulated your skin to take on a new glow. This should become a part of your daily hygiene, even after this cleansing program.

Instructions: Brush the skin for five minutes in all directions over the body except the face. Brush first thing in the morning, before you shower or bathe.

Fresh Vegetable Juices

These are important during your cleansing program. Drink the vegetable juice as soon after juicing as possible, since raw juices will lose their enzyme value quickly. If you do not have a home juicer, make your health food store a daily stop for raw juices. Some health food stores will make the juice fresh while you wait.

Instructions: Drink four ounces of vegetable juice mixed with four ounces of water, twice a day. I recommend a mixture of carrot, celery, beet, and parsley juices.

Intestinal Cleanser

This is a very important part of the cleansing program. The Intestinal Cleanser is a mixture of herbs that scrubs and cleanses both the small intestine and the colon (large intestine). It will remove buildup of undigested food and mucous that may be lining the digestive and elimination system.

Instructions: Take six Intestinal Cleanser caplets three times a day before meals.

KB-11 Tea

This is an excellent herbal combination to assist the kidneys in their function. It helps reduce water retention and aids in the elimination of uric acid and toxicity in very overworked kidneys.

Instructions: Drink one cup daily during the cleansing program.

Pau D'Arco Tea

This tea is made from tree bark imported from South America, where it has been in use for centuries. It has only recently received recognition in this country as a powerful healing tea and safe, natural antibiotic. It is very effective in reducing congestion throughout the lymph system as well as the lungs. It also helps clear mucous and acid buildup in the body. Pau D'Arco tea is a powerful aid for the immune system.

Instructions: Add one heaping tablespoon of Pau D'Arco tea bark to one quart of water. Bring to a boil and then simmer for 20 minutes. Strain off the bark, allow the tea to cool, and refrigerate. Drink eight ounces daily, hot or cold. You should continue to drink this tea after completing the cleansing program; make it a regular part of your diet.

Four-Day Cleansing Program

Day 1: Begin all products including Bilax tablets. Follow the schedule on page 56.

Day 2: Colon cleansing treatment. Continue with all products and Bilax tablets.

Day 3: Colon cleansing treatment. Continue with all products and Bilax tablets.

Day 4: Colon cleansing treatment. Use products up to the time of treatment. After the treatment discontinue use of the Intestinal Cleanser, apple cider vinegar drink, KB-11 Tea, castor oil packs, and Bilax tablets.

Seven-Day Colon Cleansing Program

Day 1:   Begin all products, including Bilax tablets. Follow the schedule below.

Day 2:   Colon cleansing treatment. Continue with all products, including Bilax tablets.

Day 3:   Colon cleansing treatment. Continue with all products, but do not take Bilax tablets.

Day 4:   Continue with all products, including Bilax tablets.

Day 5:   Colon cleansing treatment. Continue with all products, but do not take Bilax tablets.

Day 6:   Continue with all products, including Bilax tablets.

Day 7:   Colon cleansing treatment. Use products up to the time of treatment. After the treatment discontinue use of the intestinal cleanser, apple cider vinegar drink, KB-11 Tea, castor oil packs, and Bilax tablets.

Suggested Time Schedule

7:00 a.m.   **Two DDS-1 Acidophilus** capsules with water only

Five Minutes Skin Brushing, then shower or bathe

7:15 a.m.   **Intestinal Cleanser** (six caplets)

Apple Cider Vinegar Drink (one tablespoon apple cider vinegar in eight ounces of hot water; add one teaspoon maple syrup if desired)

Glass of Water (eight ounces)

8:00 a.m.   **Pau D'Arco Tea** (eight ounces)

12:00 noon   **Vegetable Juice** (four ounces of juice and four ounces of water)

1:00 p.m.	**Intestinal Cleanser** (six caplets)
	Apple Cider Vinegar Drink
	Glass of Water
3:00 p.m.	**KB-11 Tea** (eight ounces)
4:00 p.m.	**Vegetable Juice**
6:00 p.m.	**Dr. Jensen's Broth** (one teaspoon of broth in eight ounces of hot water)
8:00 p.m.	**Intestinal Cleanser** (six caplets)
	Apple Cider Vinegar Drink
	Glass of Water
8:30 p.m.	**Castor Oil Pack**
10:00 p.m.	**Bedtime**
	Two DDS-1 Acidophilus capsules with water
	On evenings before colon cleansings take **two Bilax** tablets before retiring.

Products Needed for the Colon Cleansing Program

You can order a kit containing most of the products you will need for this cleansing program by sending the order form on page 183. Allow two weeks for delivery.

All other products needed for this program can be purchased either at a drugstore or health food store.

Products Supplied in Kit
DDS-1 Acidophilus

Pau D'Arco Tea

Intestinal Cleanser

Dr. Jensen's Broth

Bilax Tablets

Castor Oil

Flannel Cloth (for castor oil application)

Dry Skin Brush

KB-11 Tea

Products to Purchase at a Drugstore
Heating Pad

Products to Purchase at a Health Food Store
Apple Cider Vinegar (Hain's or Westbrae brands only)

Raw Apple Juice

Fresh Vegetable Juices

Pure Maple Syrup (optional)

Large Plastic Garbage Bags (grocery store)

Ending Your Colon Cleansing Program

Congratulations! You have completed your Four- or Seven-Day Colon Cleansing Program! Now that you have given your digestive and elimination systems a well-earned cleansing and rest, you are going to begin eating. Hopefully, you're feeling terrific. Here comes your first food test: ending your program properly by gradually introducing solid foods to your body. The key thought to remember is moderation!

Applied to breaking a fast, this means consuming small quantities of food for the next few days.

Remember, any one can fast, but it takes wisdom to end a fast properly and not sabotage the good results achieved from this program. You can easily undo what you've done if you overeat at this time.

After your last colon cleansing, stop using the following products:

Intestinal Cleanser

Apple Cider Vinegar Drink

KB-11 Tea

Castor Oil Packs

Bilax Tablets

All the other products can be continued. I recommend that you continue drinking one cup of Pau D'Arco Tea daily and take two DDS-1 Acidophilus capsules with water first thing in the morning and just before bedtime for 30 days. Continue Bernard Jensen's Broth as desired. Have a glass of fresh vegetable juice daily; there's no better way to get concentrated nutrition.

Try to avoid orange, pineapple, and grapefruit juices; they are hard on the kidneys and high in acids.

Dry brush your skin every day; five minutes brushing before bathing in the morning will make your skin glow with health.

Food Time

First Day

Breakfast: It's best to end your fast with a specially chosen fruit on the day after your last colon cleansing. Pre-select the fruit a day or so before, so it is ready and ripe for your first breakfast. Try to select an organic fruit if possible. The best choice of fruit to end your fast is papaya. The next best choices (in order of preference) are pear, peach, plum, apple, grapes, watermelon, or any fruit in season (no citrus). Be sure to eat only one fruit.

After eating the fruit, you will find that your taste buds have been aroused and you will probably feel like eating more. Don't! Don't try to satisfy your appetite with this meal; it won't work. After a cleansing program, the body assimilates food at a faster rate so you won't get that "full-up" feeling.

Lunch: Have your lunch in the early afternoon. Try a small mixed-green salad, such as lettuce (not iceberg), sprouts, tomatoes, celery, carrots, and cucumber. Don't use salad dressing and don't have a second helping. Squeeze a lemon on your salad if desired.

Dinner: Have another small vegetable salad or another fruit (do not mix fruit and vegetables). Try to eat this meal before 7:00 p.m.

Snacks: Have vegetable juice drinks, Bernard Jensen's Broth, or herbal teas in between meals if desired.

Second Day

You may begin any vitamin and mineral supplements you were taking prior to the cleansing program.

Breakfast: Fruit salad with or without yogurt (goat yogurt, preferably).

Lunch: Mixed vegetable salad; add some protein, such as avocado or tofu. A salad dressing is fine with this salad.

Dinner: Lightly steamed vegetables with brown rice or millet (moderate portions).

Third to Seventh Day

Continue eating salads, steamed vegetables, grains, fruits, and yogurt (goat preferred).

In the weeks following your cleansing, try cutting down on the size of your meals. Your body will feel better if you consume less food. Don't try to achieve the "full-up" feeling when eating. Don't eat late in the evening or, if you must, make it a light meal, such as a fruit salad.

Consider how much food you're eating and whether your food combinations are good. Continue to use the recommended products from your cleansing program (Pau D'Arco Tea, DDS-1 Acidophilus, Bernard Jensen's Broth, fresh vegetable juices).

Repeat this cleansing program within three months.

CHAPTER 5

Lactobacillus Acidophilus: The Well-kept Secret

Lactobacillus Acidophilus: The Friendly Bacteria

Lactobacillus acidophilus is a healthful bacteria that lives in the colon. It inhibits the growth of disease-causing bacteria and is essential for normal digestion.

The routine use of antibiotics as medicine and the hidden consumption of antibiotics in meat, poultry, and dairy products destroys the natural, healthful bacteria your body needs to protect itself.

Every year in the United States over 35 million pounds of antibiotics are produced and their consumption is divided between livestock, poultry, and humans. Further, diets low in fiber and with few fresh, whole foods—and high in sugars, flours, fat, alcohol, or coffee—destroy *L. acidophilus* and encourage the growth of unfriendly putrefactive bacteria in the colon. This unfavorable shift in bacterial forms leaves you open to numerous kinds of infection and digestive distress.

L. acidophilus is a living food with unique health-giving properties. It has long been known to enhance digestion and nutrient absorption. It inhibits the growth of unfriendly bacteria, improves bowel regularity, and enhances natural immunity. *L. acidophilus* helps normalize blood cholesterol levels and even sweetens the breath.

Lactobacillus Acidophilus History

by Keith W. Sehnert, M.D.

Lactobacilli have been used in food preparation by nearly all of humankind. The Russians and Bulgarians prepared yogurt, the Danes and Germans made cheese, and the Japanese developed their miso.

In 1908, the Russian scientist Metchnikoff wrote that yogurt was the "elixir of life." He advanced the theory that yogurt could counteract the "putrefactive bacteria" in the large intestine that caused disease and shortened life. Metchnikoff reasoned that people in the Caucasus area around the Black Sea lived such long and healthy lives because of the great amount of lactobacillus they ate in their food.

In 1986, the British nutritionist K. W. Heaton reported in the *Journal of the Royal Society of Medicine* about the Asian people from Gujarat. When these Indians, primarily of the Hindu faith, immigrate to London they develop a variety of nutritional problems. These people have traditionally eaten kefir, a yogurtlike food fermented by lactobacillus. Heaton also noted that in India they eat imperfectly washed vegetables that are likely covered with lactobacillus from the soil in their gardens. When these people move to England, they eat well-washed British vegetables purchased from the local greengrocer. As time passes and the Indians become "more British" they begin eating an "endless variety of sugary foods and drinks," stop making kefir, and over a few years begin to "manifest a high prevalence of obesity, diabetes, and coronary heart disease."

A number of researchers over the years have reported on the complications resulting from the extensive use of antibiotics, emphasized the significance of a "bacterial equilibrium" in the intestinal tract, and observed the favorable influence of certain lactobacilli in counteracting the overgrowth of pathogenic organisms in the intestinal flora. Digestive disorders, including diarrhea, constipation, irritable colon and colitis, have been relieved by the administration of lactobacillus. During 1950-60, some studies were conducted to compare *L. acidophilus* with neomycin sulfate to combat *E. coli* infection. *L. acidophilus* proved to be 97 percent effective as neomycin sulfate in combating *E. coli* infection.

Lactobacillus Uses

During the nearly eight decades that marked the time between Metchnikoff and Heaton, much was learned about the Lactobacillus *family*. I emphasize the word "family" because the term "Lactobacillus" is a family name for a whole group of bacteria. They are described in bacteriology books as gram-positive, monmotile rods that ferment carbohydrates with the production of lactic acid and gas (mostly carbon dioxide). These are the bacteria that give the bubbles to champagne, the holes in Swiss cheese, and are the culprits that cause tooth decay.

Like persons with, for example, the family name of Smith, Lactobacilli have individual names and various jobs. The Smiths I know have Tom who is a banker and John who is a recreation director. The "clan" Lactobacillus has less common names and occupations. Casea makes cheese, Bulgaricus specializes in yogurt, and Fermentum turns grape juice into wine. There are many others, including the one we're interested in, Acidophilus and its special strain, DDS-1.

Not All Lactobacilli Are the Same

Although the claims and labels may look the same for lactobacillus products, the fact is they are not the same. As a result of my studies, I've decided to use DDS-1 Acidophilus because of its stability, potency effectiveness, and lower cost.

Therapeutic Effects of DDS-1

Studies conducted by scientists at the University of Nebraska and Michigan State University have shown that DDS-1 Acidophilus provides several therapeutic effects. It has specific actions including the ability to make a natural antibiotic, acidiophilin, and forms lactic acid and hydrogen peroxide.

Acidiophilin, the antibiotic, is active against a wide variety of gram-positive and gram-negative bacteria, such as *Streptococcus faecalis*, *Staphylococcus aureus*, and *Escherichea coli*, plus a host of others.

Acidophilin has also been found to retard the growth of *Candida albicans* in the laboratory. It should be noted that yogurt has long been used as a folk remedy for vaginitis. Lactobacillus organisms are normal constituents of vaginal flora. They contribute to the maintenance of the acid pH by fermenting glycogen in the mucous to lactic acid.

Nutritional Effects

In addition to the specific therapeutic effects of DDS-1, lactobacilli in general help produce B vitamins (folic acid, niacin, riboflavin, B_{12}, B_6, and pantothenic acid); aid in predigestion of proteins and formation of free amino acids; help predigest lactose (which assists people with lactose intolerance due to lack of intestinal lactase and beta-galactosidase enzymes); and have anticholesteremic and antilipedemic effects.

Miscellaneous Actions

Epidemological studies show that the ingestion of cultured dairy products may reduce the risk of colon cancer. This action is thought to be due to the effects of *L. acidophilus* on fecal enzyme activity such as beta-glucuronidase and nitro-redyctase, which change procarcinogens (cancer causing chemicals) into less harmful substances.

Comparison of Commercial Products

After a review of the many lactobacillus products, I agree with other experts that there are three criteria for consumers to consider:

1. Benefits associated with one particular strain may not necessarily apply to other strains of the same organism.

2. Commercial preparations shown to be effective in the laboratory may not contain sufficient numbers of living organisms to be of any clinical benefit.

3. Lactobacilli are fastidious in growth and metabolism, and are thus markedly affected by alcohol, antibiotic, and dietary components.

In an excellent review article, Hangee-Bauer noted that "Unfortunately, little data is available for comparing specific products, and many problems exist: many yogurts do not contain viable organisms (due to long shelf time and other factors) and products with even small amounts of glucose or sugar in them can inhibit the growth of lactobacilli for as long as three days."

While University of Nebraska researchers and others have conducted extensive studies on DDS-1 Acidophilus, U.A.S. Laboratories has developed unique manufacturing methods. These produce DDS-1 on a rice starch base and avoid corn, soy, whey, lactose, and preservatives. U.A.S. has marketed this potent, stable, and effective strain since 1979. It is the most extensively researched commercial strain available.

Each DDS-1 Acidophilus capsule contains more than one billion viable *L. acidophilus* organisms according to studies by a respected reference laboratory, A & L Midwest Agricultural Laboratories, 13611 "B" Street, Omaha, NE 68114.

General Summary of DDS-1 Advantages

When the technical and research data on DDS-1 were reviewed recently, these benefits were reported:

1. **Vitamin production:** DDS-1 is capable of producing vitamins while many other lactobacilli on the market require B vitamins for growth. The B-complex vitamins synthesized are niacin, pantothenic acid, pyrodoxine, biotin, B_6, B_{12}, and folic acid.

2. **Lactose intolerance:** Deficiency of lactase enzyme results in the inefficient digestion of lactose (milk sugar), a condition called lactose intolerance. DDS-1 produces lactase enzyme, which helps digest lactose.

3. **Food digestion:** DDS-1 produces enzymes that help digest food and decrease bloating.

4. **Reduces cholesterol:** DDS-1 possesses anticholesteremic and antilipidemic factors. Several studies show significant reduction of serum cholesterol levels after supplementation with DDS-1.

5. **Prevents bad breath:** Colonization of putrefying bacteria in large numbers in the throat, tongue, and mouth causes halitosis (bad breath). When these putrefying bacteria are dominant in the intestine, they produce objectionable gases. DDS-1 helps keep those putrefying bacteria in check, thus helping prevent bad breath.

6. **Natural antibiotic:** DDS-1 is known to produce acidophilin, a natural antibiotic, which has been shown to possess (in vitro) a wide range of antimicrobial activity against common foodborne pathogens. The following organisms can be inhibited by acidophilin:

   Bacillus subtilis

   Bacillus cereus

   Bacillus stearothermophilus

   Streptococcus faecalis var. liquifaciens

   Streptococcus lactis

Lactobacillus lactis

Lactobacillus casei

Lactobacillus plantarum

Lactobacillus leichmannii

Sarcina lutea

Serratia marcescens

Proteus vulgaris

Escherichia coli

Salmonella typhosa

Salmonella schottmuelleri

Shigella dysenteriae

Shigella paradysenteriae

Pseudomonas fluorescens

Pseudomonas aeruginosa

Staphylococcus aureus

Klebsiella pneumoniae

Vibrio comma

7. **Antiviral effects:** *L. acidophilus* can inactivate many different viruses.

8. **Cold-sore management:** Cold sores (fever blisters) are caused by *Herpes simplex*, which often can be prevented or even cured by supplementation with DDS-1.

9. **Inhibition of *Candida albicans*:** Inhibition of this common yeast is possible with supplementation of DDS-1 and this has been confirmed by clinical studies.

10. **Anticarcinogenic effects:** Studies at Sloan Kettering Institute for Cancer Research and the University of Nebraska show DDS-1 to possess definite antitumor activity and to have inhibited tumor proliferation by 41 percent.

Conclusions

Persons who are heading to a health food store to buy a lactobacillus product should remember the advice once given by a Roman philosopher: "caveat emptor" or "buyer beware." The labels and promotional literature of many products claim a high bacterial count only because they do not use pure *Lactobacillis acidophilus* and raise their count by using *other* bacteria in the mixture. Others have a low count on lactobacillus organism because they were not properly stored after manufacturing was completed. Still others get around the truth by variations in dosage. Instead of the two capsules per day recommended for DDS-1, they advise "two to four capsules, two to four times per day," which is 16 capsules for a comparable dose! Other firms may promote their product by referring to DDS-1 research—not their *own*! Ask the druggist or store manager to show you technical data on the product. Read it carefully. You will discover what I found: *not all lactobacilli are the same!*

Note

DDS-1 Acidophilus has been developed in a rice starch base. No dairy, corn, soy, or preservatives have been added. It is also important to know that many acidophilus products in the market do not colonize in the colon. DDS-1 Acidophilus is acid-resistant and implants in the colon.

An order form for DDS-1 Acidophilus capsules is on page 185.

Reprinted by permission of Keith W. Sehnert, M.D.

CHAPTER 6

Candida Albicans Overgrowth: The Quiet Epidemic

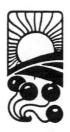

How to Fight Candida and Survive

by Tom Valentine

"Untreated systemic candidiasis has a mortality rate approaching 100 percent. Delay in treatment is dangerous and will almost certainly end in death of the patient."

That telling statement was written by Dr. Richard Hurley of London in a medical paper.

"When tests are done on estrogen levels, thyroid levels, or other hormone levels and people are suffering from these symptoms (candidiasis), the hormones are there in the bloodstream, but they are not activating any response."

C. Orian Truss, M.D., the leading authority on chronic candidiasis, made the above statement when describing the insidious attacks the common fungus *Candida albicans* makes on human endocrine and immune systems.

Hormones are essential to our health, and our bloodstream must be literally crawling with them in order for our bodies to operate in a normal, balanced manner. Candidiasis taking hold of the endocrine system and imbalancing hormonal function is a major health problem that has yet to be fully diagnosed and understood by the mainstream medical establishment.

Candidiasis has a way of disarming our immune systems, and if that sounds like AIDS (Acquired Immune Deficiency Syndrome) to you, join the club that is seeing more links between the two deadly infections than the establishment cares to admit.

There is strong sentiment among Americans that the drug-monopolized, bureaucratically controlled medical establishment has failed them. More and more people are looking back at their medical histories and seeing that what they had previously suffered was undiagnosed chronic candidiasis.

A Natural War

There is a war going on inside every one of us. It's a war between natural microbes in our systems, and we have been losing for decades because of our medical establishment's combination of arrogance and ignorance, or criminal neglect, or both.

Our vital endocrine system (thyroid, thymus, parathyroid, pineal, pituitary, adrenal, pancreas, ovaries, testes) should not be infected by naturally occurring intestinal fungus. But, it is—with devastating, generally undiagnosed effects.

The drug industry lock on medical technology and education has helped create an arrogant ignorance within the profession that has been further enhanced by monopolistic bureaucracy. To now be told by courageous researchers, defying established dogma, that the "wonder drugs" of the past have unleashed an epidemic of immune-destroying chronic candidiasis, calls for charges of criminal negligence.

Why do a few independent researchers have to put their reputations on the line and "discover" that the common yeast, *Candida albicans*, is wreaking havoc with our national health? Why didn't the great institutions learn this natural fact decades ago? Hippocrates, the father of medicine, noted the common candida-caused infections of vaginitis and oral thrush more than 1500 years before the microscope.

However, to point out the flaws and establish blame does not solve the problem. What's done is done. Now the people must act to help themselves, and at the same time to force political changes that will result in a revamping of the medical bureaucracy.

The big problem of the moment is to stop candidiasis before it stops us. Candida has the upper hand right now because millions remain in ignorance and joyously starve their own systems while feeding the fungus.

AIDS—Plus

How bad is it? Let's look at the latest from the AIDS front. Even those who don't know about candida have heard about AIDS. There's no link between the two, you say. One is virally caused, the other is a mold, you say.

Robert S. Mendelsohn, who publishes *The People's Doctor*, a monthly newsletter (P.O. Box 982, Evanston, IL 60204), pointed out that the latest bulletin from the medical establishment (*FDA Drug Bulletin*) places some forms of candidiasis in a category now called "lesser AIDS."

In his February 1985 newsletter, the doctor who points out the flaws in his profession for the benefit of the people, wrote:

This new, expanded definition of AIDS, of course, raises a new set of questions. The government doctors have reassured us that no cases of AIDS have been found in members of families of AIDS victims. However, with this new definition, those old studies become worthless until the families are restudied for these additional diseases.

Perhaps even more importantly, the HTLV-III test, like any other laboratory test, produces not only false-positive results, but false-negatives. Therefore, if a person has one of these diseases now listed under the AIDS umbrella, how do the doctors know that, even in the absence of a positive AIDS blood test, the patient does not have AIDS?

In case you aren't confused enough by now, the FDA Drug Bulletin *states: "In addition, idiopathic thrombocytopenia (a blood condition) is probably associated with the HTLV-III infection, as are a variety of non-life threatening fungal and bacterial infectious processes. . . ." The doctors call these manifestations lesser AIDS.*

So now we have AIDS, ARC (AIDS related complex) and lesser AIDS. When it comes to the causes of AIDS or its symptomatology, do any researchers or government doctors really know what they're talking about?

Based on the in-depth research of Dr. Truss, the listing of "pulmonary candidiasis" (yeast infection of the breathing system) as being among the "lesser AIDS" complex is more than a little scary.

Dr. Truss, a Birmingham, Alabama, physician, wrote *The Missing Diagnosis*, and is considered the world's top authority on chronic candidiasis—which is much more than a simple yeast infection, even though the same critter is involved.

Dr. Truss has cured patients of debilitating conditions, which had virtually wrecked their lives, by discovering that the patients were not "neurotic," nor did they need "psychiatry" simply because medicine could not correctly diagnose their chronic candidiasis.

Candida Albicans

Candida albicans is among the most common of yeasts or molds or fungi. It may be found in every human intestinal tract from the mouth (especially fond of dentures) to the anus, and in every vagina. Normally, the fungus is kept under control by friendly bacteria, such as *Lactobacillus acidophilus*, so it poses no threat to health.

Many times we hear a person say, "Oh, that's only a yeast

infection, that's not serious." This is an attitude nurtured by the establishment's attitude. Obviously a wrong attitude.

"The yeast lives in everyone," Dr. Truss told *Acres U.S.A.* "However, when it is stimulated by various factors, especially antibiotics and birth control pills, it may establish a chronic infection known as chronic candidiasis."

What happens, Dr. Truss explained, is that the yeast is not affected by the broad spectrum antibiotics, which kill off the friendly bacteria by the billions. Antibiotics are the worst, but not the only drug-induced cause for chronic candidiasis. With the friendly bacteria obliterated, the fungus overgrows its normalcy and the individual's immune system must deal with the spreading mold. "Once candida gets into other tissues and into the bloodstream, it has the ability to overcome the immune system."

That sounds a lot like AIDS, does it not?

To make matters worse, researchers at the University of Iowa recently discovered that *Candida albicans* has chameleonlike abilities to change form—making it difficult to control.

According to the *Des Moines Register*, December 30, 1985, biologists at the University of Iowa described the common fungus as "a microscopic monster capable of inflicting a wide range of torture" on patients. "Until recently, however, nobody knew candida very well. Now it appears the common yeast is a more terrible creature than anyone suspected—a Dr. Jekyll and Mr. Hyde character capable of changing its looks and personality and then changing back to its original form."

Another aspect that sounds like AIDS!

"Dr. David Soll, the University of Iowa biologist who discovered candida's quick-change capability, says it may be what allows the fungus to elude both antibiotics and the body's immune system," the article added.

It is incredible that the wonders of modern medical technology somehow overlooked this fungus until Dr. Truss

79

and others screamed so loudly they could no longer be ignored.

Now, we note, a number of financial grants are finding their way into universities as the drug monopoly scurries to cover its proverbial behind with patentable pharmacology to stop the spread of this common critter that drugs helped unleash in the first place.

In our technical sophistication, arrogant mankind seems to forget that "it isn't wise to fool nature."

Among the data from the study was the discovery that a particular drug, ketoconazole, does not work for "immuno-suppressed patients." Immunosuppression is curious logic, unless you think you're smarter than nature.

According to Dr. Truss:

An immunosuppressant drug is a drug that suppresses or weakens the immune defenses of the body. Many symptoms of illness are actually due to the inflammation that results when the white blood cells respond in defense against some injurious or potentially dangerous factor.

Symptoms may be due to the body's defensive response to a germ, rather than to the germ itself. A sore throat or the inflamed tissues of the nose and throat characteristic of the common cold are familiar examples. Even when the inflammation is not clearly related to an infectious agent, for example rheumatoid arthritis, it is quite likely that most of the symptoms result from the immune response to an as yet undiscovered cause of the disease.

Since inflammation is distressing to patients, the medical profession happily accepted from the drug manufacturers a group of drugs designed to suppress the immune system and make the inflammation go away.

"Unfortunately," Dr. Truss added, "it is not possible to suppress just one manifestation of immunity without impairing the entire immune response."

Cortisone-type hormone drugs are the most commonly used immunosuppressives, and Dr. Truss lists them among the major causes of the epidemic spread of chronic candidiasis.

Contributing Factors

Let's add it all up. Our society is crawling with pollutants that enhance candida and clobber us. Our food is refined, additivized, and chemicalized, and then so loaded with sugars and starch that we feed candida very happily—beer-belly bloat is an obvious "sign" of candidiasis.

There is also the "health food" known as brewer's yeast. Most B vitamins come in brewer's yeast bases. It serves to strengthen candida.

Infants on the mother's breast, Dr. Truss said, have a strong *Lactobacillus acidophilus* count and candidiasis is not normally seen. But once off the breast, candidiasis will show up in a hurry—it's known as diaper rash.

The critter is chasing us from cradle to grave—gleefully. One doctor noted that "the living human is nothing more than organic matter that needs recycling to *Candida albicans*."

Antibiotics are everywhere in our society—in meats and poultry, in the hands of every pediatrician, even over-the-counter. Add the technical wonders of cortisone and birth control pills and you have an epidemic.

The symptoms of chronic candidiasis include:

Central nervous system disorders: depression, anxiety, irrational irritability, lethargy, fatigue, agitation, inability to concentrate, memory loss, and headaches, including migraines.

Intestinal disorders: bloating, diarrhea, constipation, heartburn, gastritis, indigestion, and colitis.

Allergic manifestations: severe chemical and food sensitivities, asthma, acne, hives, sinusitis, hay fever, skin rashes, earaches, and possibly psoriasis.

In children there is hyperactivity, irritability, learning problems, poor appetite, and erratic sleep patterns as well as the other symptoms. One of the most used, if not the most used, medical techniques today is the ear-tube operation for children.

What can you do to protect yourself?

Doctors are prescribing nystatin, but as with all drugs there are drawbacks and side effects. Besides, there is evidence that when the nystatin is halted, the yeast comes back with a vengeance. Herbalists suggest garlic, but doctors say it is ineffective.

There are a number of independent physicians striving to cope with the pandemic, which is still largely unrecognized by the medical establishment. The best way to avoid or overcome chronic candidiasis is with a careful dietary program and the reestablishment of friendly bacteria.

Nothing fights *Candida albicans*, in all its forms, better than *Lactobacillus acidophilus*, especially the DDS-1 strain developed at the University of Nebraska.

Recovery

It takes a long time to recover balance and health. We didn't wreck our systems overnight, and we can't recover overnight.

The Yeast Connection, a book by William Crook, M.D., is available in most bookstores and through *Acres U.S.A.* It is a valuable weapon in this war. *The Missing Diagnosis*, by Dr. Orian Truss is also available. Also, HEALTHEXCEL (509-996-2131) tailors an individual nutritional program that deals with candida effectively. The object is to avoid yeast-feeding foods and feed your own metabolic system.

This reporter is also testing on himself and his family members a low-cost, nontoxic, nonmonopolizable substance that could turn the tide in this war against parasites of both varieties—mold and man.

Reprinted by permission of Tom Valentine from Acres U.S.A., *June 1986.*

Candida Albicans Overgrowth

by William Wolcott

What Is Candida?

We all live in a virtual sea of microorganisms—bacteria, viruses, fungi, and so forth. These microbes can reside in the throat, mouth, nose, intestinal tract, or almost anywhere; they are as much a part of our bodies as the food we eat. Usually, these microorganisms do not cause illness, unless our resistance becomes lowered.

Candida albicans is a yeast that lives in the mouth, throat, intestines, and genitourinary tract of most humans and is usually considered to be a normal part of the bowel flora (the organisms that coexist with us in our lower digestive tract). Candida is actually a member of a broader classification of organisms known as fungi.

Traditionally, fungi are considered plants, but they contain no chlorophyll and cannot make their own food. Fungi tend to inhabit cool to tropical climates and are found in the air we breathe as well as in moist, shady soil, water, manure, dead leaves, fruit, leftover food, and in a wide variety of places and circumstances.

How Do You Get Candida?

Candida albicans prefers people. Candida enters newborn infants during or shortly after birth. Usually, the growth of the yeast is kept in check by the infant's immune system and thus produces no overt symptoms. But, should the immune response weaken, the condition known as oral thrush can occur as a result. By six months of age, 90 percent of all babies test positive for candida. And by adulthood, virtually all humans play host to *Candida albicans* and are thus engaged in a lifelong relationship.

Candida coexists in our bodies with many species of bacteria in a competitive balance. Other bacteria act in part to keep candida growth in check, unless that balance is upset. When health is present, the immune system keeps candida proliferation under control; but when immune response is weakened, candida growth can proceed unhindered. It is an "opportunistic organism," one which, when given the opportunity, will attempt to colonize all bodily tissues. The uncontrolled growth of candida is known as *candida overgrowth*.

Causes of Candida Overgrowth

It is well known that the immune system is highly dependent on the proper biochemical balance in the body. Unfortunately, there are many factors in our modern society that can upset the ecological balance of the body, weaken the immune system, and thus allow the yeast to overgrow. Many physicians cognizant of candida report that 50 to 70 percent of their patients have candida overgrowth. These seemingly epidemic proportions are attributed to the general decline of vitality—specifically in relation to the immune system—in our society as a result of generations of suboptimal diets and other associated factors of drug and chemical exposures.

Traditional foods have been notably replaced by severely altered foods from a multitude of "modern" treatment methods in growing, processing, and packaging. Heating, pressurizing, preserving, refining, stabilizing, and even creating synthetic foods have all resulted in the considerable alteration of nutrient intake from what had been the previous norm for thousands of years.

Radical alterations in life-style that have accompanied rapid modernization in the twentieth century have brought unforeseen and previously uncommon stresses that the human body must now cope with in its efforts at adaptation. Pollution of our air, water, and food; new medications and drugs, both prescription and nonprescription; alcohol; tobacco; high carbohydrate and sugar intake in our diets; chronic food and chemical allergies—all put a considerable strain on the immune system.

There is a growing awareness of the link between major illnesses, such as cancer, diabetes, heart disease, and schizophrenia to diet and environmental factors and their adverse affects on the immune system. *Candida albicans*, usually a benign yeast held in check by the immune system, proliferates when the immune system becomes unbalanced, compromised, or weakened. The major risk factors that may predispose you to the proliferation of candida are the following:

Antibiotics and Sulfa Drugs. Probably the chief culprit of all, antibiotics kill all bacteria; they do not distinguish the good from the bad. Antibiotics kill the "good" flora that normally keep candida under control. This allows for the unchecked growth of candida in the intestinal tract.

It is normally difficult to recover a yeast culture from bodily surfaces. However, after 48 hours of taking tetracycline, yeast can be cultivated easily from anyone. The prevalence today of candida may be most directly related to the widespread societal exposure to antibiotics—from prescriptions for colds, infections, acne, and from additional consumption of antibiotic-treated foods, such as meats, dairy, poultry, and eggs.

The rapid and direct proliferation of the yeast following antibiotic use strongly suggests that the problem of candida is one that stems from an inner state of imbalance, rather than from an outside attack by a microbe or disease.

Steroid Hormones and Immunosuppressant Drugs. These drugs, such as cortisone, treat severe allergic problems by paralyzing the immune system's ability to react.

Pregnancy, Multiple Pregnancies, or Birth Control Pills. These upset the body's hormonal balance.

Improper Diet. Diets high in carbohydrate and sugar intake, yeast and yeast products, and molds and fermented foods encourage candida overgrowth.

Environmental Hazards. Prolonged exposure to environmental molds as well as an increasing number of chemicals in food, water and air, including petrochemicals, formaldehyde, perfumes, cleaning fluids, insecticides, tobacco, and other indoor and outdoor pollutants, make the system more susceptible to yeast imbalance.

Once begun, candida overgrowth can result in a self-perpetuating, negative cycle if not recognized and treated appropriately. Large numbers of yeast germs can weaken the immune system, which normally protects the body from harmful invaders. The immune system may concurrently be adversely affected by poor nutrition and heavy exposure to environmental toxins.

The resulting lowered resistance may not only cause an overall sense of ill health, but may allow for the development of respiratory, digestive, and other systemic symptoms. People may also become predisposed to developing sensitivities to foods and chemicals in the environment. Such "allergies" may in turn cause the membranes of the nose, throat, ear, bladder, and intestinal tract to swell and develop infection.

Such conditions may lead the physician to prescribe a "broad spectrum" antibiotic that may then further promote the overgrowth of candida and strengthen the existing negative chain of events, leading to further stress on the immune system and increased candida-related problems.

What Are the Signs of Candida Infections?

The result of heightened candida overgrowth is a list of adverse symptoms of considerable length. Basically, the characteristics of candida overgrowth fall under three categories: those affecting the gastrointestinal and genitourinary tracts; allergic responses; and mental/emotional manifestations.

Initially, the signs will show near the sights of the original yeast colonies. Most often, the first signs are seen in conditions such as nasal congestion and discharge, nasal itching, blisters in the mouth, sore or dry throat, abdominal pain, belching, bloating, heartburn, constipation, diarrhea, rectal burning or itching, vaginal discharge, vaginal itching or burning, increasingly worsening symptoms of PMS (premenstrual syndrome), prostatitis, impotence, frequent urination, burning on urination, and bladder infections.

But, if the immune system remains weak long enough, candida can spread to all parts of the body causing an additional plethora of problems. Most commonly these include the gastrointestinal tract with all manner of digestive disturbances, food allergies, sensitivities, and cravings for sweets; central nervous system disorders, such as fatigue, drowsiness, uncoordination, lack of concentration, dizziness, headaches; musculoskeletal problems involving joint swelling, migrating aches and pains, and arthritis; hormonal disruptions, such as menstrual irregularities; problems with eyes, ears, and the respiratory system, such as spots in front of the eyes, failing vision, burning or tearing eyes, ear pain and deafness, bad breath, coughing, wheezing, asthma, and hay fever; skin problems, such as hives, rashes, eczema, psoriasis, dry skin, and chronic fungal infections, such as athlete's foot, ringworm, and fingernail/toenail infections; impairment of the circulatory system, such as cold hands and feet, numbness and tingling sensations; and aberrations in personality and behavior, such as anxiety, depression, hyperirritability, and mood swings.

In addition, 79 different toxic products are known to be released by candida, which places a considerable burden on the immune system. These toxins get into the bloodstream and travel to all parts of the body where they may cause a host of adverse symptoms.

In candida overgrowth, the yeast colonies can dig deep into intestinal walls, damaging the bowel wall in their colonization. Candida can also attack the immune system, causing suppressor cell disease, in which the immune system produces antibodies to everything at the slightest provocation, resulting in extreme sensitivities. Finally, candida overgrowth can be dangerous if not controlled. The persistent, constant challenge to the immune system by an ever-increasing, long-term overgrowth of candida can eventually serve to wear down the immune system and cause a seriously weakened capacity for resistance to disease.

Women are more likely to get candida overgrowth than are men. This is related to the female sex hormone progesterone, which is elevated in the last half of the menstrual cycle. Progesterone increases the amount of glycogen (animal starch, easily converted to sugar) in the vaginal tissues, which provides an ideal growth medium for candida. Progesterone levels also elevate during pregnancy. Men are affected less frequently but are by no means invulnerable.

How Do You Know You Have Candida?

Currently, diagnosis is primarily clinical. Since almost all people have candida in their bodies, tests for its presence are useless; confirmation of overgrowth is very difficult through laboratory tests. And, since candida paralyzes the immune system against it, allergy tests to determine the system's reaction to it are also ineffectual.

Furthermore, the results of the yeast imbalance—the combined effects of different hormones, poisons generated and released by the yeast into the bloodstream, and the confusion created in the immune system—produce a wide variety of symptoms that are seemingly unrelated (such as wheezing, depression, and fungus infection under fingernails). Thus, it is difficult to make a definite diagnosis from any specific pattern of signs and symptoms.

Currently, the best test still seems to be the therapeutic trial. A joint decision is usually made by the physician and the patient after analyzing the individual's case history. (Many physicians regard vaginal yeast infections as the most reliable indicator of candida overgrowth in women, for example.) A tentative diagnosis is made, based on the patient's history of symptoms in relation to any known possible predisposing factors, which is then proven true or false by the way the patient responds to the therapy.

Many physicians now believe that a clinical trial for candida overgrowth is of so little risk and expense that it should be considered in any chronic illness. One clinical trial you may try for five days is to avoid eating certain foods that are known to facilitate the growth of yeast. Such foods include the following:

Sugar and Carbohydrates found in all sweetened foods, including honey, molasses, sorghum, maple syrup, sugar, fructose, maltose, and dextrose. Also, fresh fruits, dried fruits, and fresh, frozen, and canned juices should be eliminated, as well as soda pop.

Yeast Products, such as beer, wine, saki, liquor, bread, natural B vitamins, and brewer's yeast.

Fermented and Mold Foods, such as mushrooms, cheese, vinegar, mustard, catsup, relish and other condiments made with vinegar, sour cream, buttermilk, tofu, soy sauce, and miso.

After eliminating these foods for five days, try adding them back into your diet in large quantities. By observing how you feel while off these foods, in comparison to any adverse affects experienced when going back on the foods, you may get a clue as to any possible yeast involvement as a causative factor for any adverse symptoms.

How Do You Get Rid of Candida Overgrowth?

Although diagnosis and supervision of treatment require a physician, the reacquisition of health and control of candida by the immune system also depends a great deal on the effort of the candida patient. Generally, treatment of candida involves four major considerations:

1. Destroying the yeast.

2. Eliminating, if possible, immunosuppressive drugs and antibiotics, or curtailing their use to only when absolutely necessary.

3. Depriving the candida of those foods on which it is nourished and flourishes.

4. Rebalancing and strengthening of the body's immune system for the restoration of proper function through dietary measures that will meet individual nutritional requirements.

To destroy candida, or "to even the odds" so to speak, a physician may prescribe a drug by the name of nystatin, or one of several available products containing nystatin. It is an antibiotic, which means that it is made by one kind of germ, such as a mold, to kill another germ, such as strep, staph, or tuberculosis.

Nystatin is an antibiotic that kills yeasts and only yeasts. It is one of the least toxic known drugs; even when large amounts are ingested, only small traces actually get into the bloodstream. The pure powdered form is generally accepted as most effective.

Nystatin and caprylic acid products are deadly to candida. Depending on the severity of candida overgrowth and the amount of the agents taken, the candida can be killed off in vast numbers in a very short period of time. As they are killed, they release substances that are toxic to the body. If this process occurs more quickly than the toxins can be cleared from the bloodstream and eliminated by the body, a temporary toxic or allergic-type reaction can occur. The technical name for this experience is a "Herxheimer reaction," more commonly referred to as "die-off."

Usually die-off lasts only a few hours, although it can last several days. It can usually be controlled almost entirely by the amount of ingestion of the agent and the rate or frequency it is taken. Signs of Herxheimer reaction can be many and varied, but generally involve such discomfort as aching, bloating, nausea, and an overall "goopy sick" feeling, or a worsening of original symptoms. Fortunately, die-off is generally short in duration, and although uncomfortable, is at least a confirmation of the presence of candida and that something good is happening.

Exercise as well as colonics and enemas are helpful in countering the adversities of die-off.

Although nystatin is very effective in killing candida, many people develop an allergic-type sensitivity to it with prolonged use. For this reason, many physicians are now considering alternatives for the job. Foremost among these is the use of products containing caprylic acid.

Caprylic acid is a natural substance, a fatty acid, that is totally lethal to candida. It is available over the counter and appears to be equal to nystatin in effectiveness. However, it is not known to produce the sensitivity side effects of the nystatin drugs. Of the caprylic acid products on the market, CAPRYSTATIN, KAPRYCIDIN-A, and ORITHRUSH-D Gargle, when used together, appear to be the most effective by virtue of their capacity to address the entire digestive tract.

Other natural aids in the fight against candida are garlic and Pau D'Arco (or Taheebo) tea, both believed to have natural fungicidal properties. Garlic is preferably taken raw, but may be effectively utilized in capsule form in a product by the name of Arizona Natural Garlic, available in most heath food stores.

At the end of this chapter is the Eight-Week Candida Overgrowth Elimination Program, which recommends products and directions for the elimination of candida overgrowth.

Proper Diet

Research has found that the immune system is highly sensitive to the proper biochemical balance in the body, which also effects the immune system's efficient functioning. A growing amount of nutritional research suggests that although everyone requires the same nutrients to maintain metabolic processes, different people need different amounts of nutrients to meet the optimal requirements of their nutritional individuality.

For these reasons, HEALTHEXCEL provides a scientific means of identifying individual nutritional requirements based on the determination of the individual's "metabolic type," i.e., the genetically determined metabolic and nutritional parameters. It is because different people have different metabolic types, and therefore different needs for nutrition, that the allopathic, symptom-treatment approach in nutrition is baseless and so often ineffective. This further explains why, nutritionally, what helps make one person feel better may have little or no effect on another, or even make a third person feel worse. Once the metabolic type is determined, a diet and supplementation program can be recommended to meet individual nutritional requirements, thus providing an ideal means of restoring proper biochemical balance.

In addition, the use of natural, live acidophilus culture, such as that found in the product DDS-1, has been found to be helpful to aid the body in restoring the proper intestinal flora balance.

Many people with candida overgrowth find it very difficult to "get off" an antifungal agent, such as nystatin or caprylic acid, without a recurrence of the problem. In lieu of such circumstances, consider the following:

- If different people have different requirements for nutrition, and
- If the immune system is highly dependent on the proper biochemical balance to function efficiently, and
- If the immune system is supposed to keep candida in check, and
- If the problem of candida overgrowth recurs when you

stop the antifungal agent, then it is possible that you are following a diet that is inappropriate for your immune system, which may in part be responsible for your body's failure to control the yeast.

Ideally, then, it is HEALTHEXCEL's recommendation that the attending physician suggest that anyone with candida overgrowth adhere to a diet that is correct for that person's metabolic type.

Unfortunately, it's not sufficient to get rid of the symptoms of candida overgrowth to the exclusion of the underlying cause of the problem: a compromised immune system. Thus, if you ignore your nutritional individuality, you may also find that although you are temporarily successful in ridding your system of candida, your success may be short-lived and you may experience a recurrence of the problem. The next logical step is to improve your overall immune efficiency by addressing your individual metabolic requirements.

Conclusion

Total elimination of yeast from the body is neither feasible nor desirable, considering that yeast are very likely beneficial to the body when a proper balance exists. Treatment of candida overgrowth does not seek the eradication of candida from the diet or the person, but rather a *restoration of the proper and balanced relationship between the person and yeast*.

Candida albicans, if uncontrolled, may indeed pose a serious threat to health and well-being. Another perspective, however, may view candida as a kind of "early warning system." Candida in a well-balanced body chemistry is merely a part of a greater environmental whole that very likely provides some benefit to the host with whom it coexists.

It is only when the body chemistry develops imbalance and the immune system is compromised as a result that overgrowth becomes a problem to be reckoned with. It is a signal to us that drugs, improper foods or other forms of distress have significantly weakened our defenses and undermined our good health. Viewed from this perspective, the presence of the early warning signals afforded us by *candida albicans* may actually allow for the avoidance of future disaster.

Reprinted by permission of William Wolcott.

Candida Albicans Self-test

Introduction

The following questionnaire was designed by William G. Crook, M.D., to be used by adults to identify their predisposition to *candida albicans* yeast infection. It is not intended as a means for diagnosis, but only as an organized system for gathering information regarding candida. If you score high on this questionnaire, you may wish to bring it to your physician's attention. Your physician may then wish to run clinical tests in order to determine whether or not you have abnormal candida growth presently occurring. Any therapy in this regard will depend on your physician's judgment.

It is not within the jurisdiction of the author to diagnose the presence of candida, nor to recommend any therapeutic action. The author recognizes this activity as the sole responsibility of the attending physician.

This material is being provided for educational and informational purposes only, in hopes that it may prove of use to you and your physician.

Instructions

Section A pertains to factors in your medical history that may promote the imbalanced growth of candida. Sections B and C are concerned with symptoms that are commonly seen in individuals with yeast-connected illnesses.

For each "Yes" answer you have in Section A, circle the Point Score in that section. At the end of the section, total your score and record it on the Total Score line. Then move to Sections B and C, and score as indicated.

Scoring

According to Dr. Crook, yeast-connected health problems are *almost certainly* present in women with scores over 180, and in men with scores over 140. (Women's scores will tend to run higher, as seven items apply exclusively to women, while only two apply exclusively to men.)

Yeast-connected health problems are *probably* present in women with scores over 120, and in men with scores over 90.

Yeast-connected health problems are *possibly* present in women with scores over 60, and in men with scores over 40.

If you feel from answering the questionnaire that you may have a candida overgrowth problem, then it is recommended that you consider doing the self-help candida overgrowth reduction program on page 104.

Section A: History

Have you taken tetracyclines (Sumycin®, Panmycin®, Vibramycin®, Minocin®, etc.) or other antibiotics for acne for one month or longer?   25

Have you at any time in your life taken other "broad-spectrum" antibiotics (ampicillin, amoxicillin, Ceclor®, Bactrim®, Septra®, Keflex®, etc.) for respiratory, urinary or other infections for two months or longer, or in shorter course, four or more times in a one-year period?   20

Have you taken a broad-spectrum antibiotic drug, even a single course?   6

Have you at any time in your life been bothered by persistent prostatitis, vaginitis or other problems affecting your reproductive organs?   25

Have you been pregnant:
    Two or more times?   5
    One time?   3

Have you taken birth control pills:
    For more than two years?   15
    For two weeks or less?   8

Have you taken prednisone, Decadron® or other cortisone-type drugs:
    For more than two weeks?   15
    For two weeks or less?   6

Does exposure to perfumes, insecticides, fabric-shop odors, and other chemicals provoke:

    Moderate or severe symptoms?   20

    Mild symptoms?   5

Are symptoms worse on damp, muggy days or in moldy places?   20

Have you had athlete's foot, ringworm, jock itch, or other chronic fungus infections of the skin or nails:

    Severe or persistent?   20

    Mild to moderate?   10

Do you crave sugar?   10

Do you crave breads?   10

Do you crave alcoholic beverages?   10

Does tobacco smoke really bother you?   10

Total Score Section A   ————

Section B: Major Symptoms

For each of your symptoms, enter the appropriate figure in the Point Score column:

If a symptom is **occasional or mild**; score 3 points.

If a symptom is **frequent and/or moderately severe**; score 6 points.

If a symptom is **severe and/or disabling**; score 9 points.

	Point Score
Fatigue or lethargy	_____
Feeling of being drained	_____
Poor memory	_____
Feeling spacey or unreal	_____
Depression	_____
Numbness, burning or tingling	_____
Muscle aches	_____
Muscle weakness or paralysis	_____
Pain and/or swelling in joints	_____
Abdominal pain	_____
Constipation	_____
Diarrhea	_____
Bloating	_____
Troublesome vaginal discharge	_____
Persistent vaginal burning or itching	_____
Prostatitis	_____
Impotence	_____
Loss of sexual desire	_____
Endometriosis	_____

Cramps and/or other menstrual irregularities ———————

Premenstrual tension (PMS)   ———————

Spots in front of eyes   ———————

Erratic vision   ———————

Total Score Section B   ———————

Section C: Other Symptoms

For each of your symptoms, enter the appropriate figure in the Point Score column:

If a symptom is **occasional or mild**; score 3 points.

If a symptom is **frequent and/or moderately severe**; score 6 points.

If a symptom is **severe and/or disabling**; score 9 points.

	Point Score
Drowsiness	_____
Irritability or jitteriness	_____
Uncoordination	_____
Inability to concentrate	_____
Frequent mood swings	_____
Headaches	_____
Dizziness/loss of balance	_____
Pressure above ears; feeling of head swelling or tingling	_____
Itching	_____
Other rashes	_____
Heartburn	_____
Indigestion	_____
Belching and intestinal gas	_____
Mucous in stools	_____
Hemorrhoids	_____
Dry mouth	_____
Rash or blisters in mouth	_____
Bad breath	_____

Joint swelling or arthritis   _____

Nasal congestion or discharge   _____

Postnasal drip   _____

Nasal twitching   _____

Sore or dry throat   _____

Cough   _____

Pain or tightness in chest   _____

Wheezing or shortness of breath _____

Urgency or urinary frequency   _____

Burning on urination   _____

Failing vision   _____

Burning or tearing of eyes   _____

Recurrent infections or fluid in ears _____

Ear pain or deafness   _____

Total Score Section C   _____

Total Score Section A   _____

Total Score Section B   _____

GRAND TOTAL SCORE   _____

Eight-Week Candida Overgrowth Elimination Program

Required Products

Each product is designed to give a specific result. Do not make any substitutions. The order form for these products is on page 186.

Arizona Natural Garlic	Antifungal and blood purifier
Caprystatin	Antifungal for lower bowel, time-release
Intestinal Cleanser	Bulking agent to help clean out candida overgrowth
Co-enzyme Q10	For the immune system
DDS-1	Acidophilus culture (always refrigerate)
Kaprycidin-A	Antifungal for stomach and upper intestines
Megavital	For immune building and nutrition
Orithrush-D Gargle	Antifungal for mouth to stomach
Pau D'Arco Tea	Antifungal
Travacid X	Digestive aid

Food Restrictions

During the eight-week program, you must eliminate foods that are known to stimulate candida growth. The foods upon which candida thrive and flourish include the following list. **Do not eat these foods!**

Sweets: Sugar, honey, molasses, syrup, sweeteners, all fruits (fresh and dried), and all fruit juices (fresh, canned or frozen). When you crave sugar, it's the candida doing the beckoning, not your system.

Molds and Fermented Foods: Cheese, sour cream, buttermilk, mushrooms, vinegar, soy sauce, cider, tofu, catsup, mustard, relish, and any pickled products. Yeast, molds, and fungi all cross-react.

Processed Meats: Processed meat with additives, breaded and pickled meats, and meats that are cured, dried, or smoked, such as ham, bacon, corned beef, pastrami, salami, hot dogs, lunch meat, and sausages. These foods are loaded with molds.

Foods Containing Yeast: Many health professionals are divided on this subject. Some feel that all yeast foods should be restricted, while others feel that nutritional yeast foods that do not contain live yeast (particularily of the candida strain) and have been cooked pose no problem and therefore can be eaten during a candida overgrowth elimination program. HEALTHEXCEL supports the opinion of those favoring the inclusion of yeast foods in the diet unless you have a past history of nutritional yeast sensitivities; in that case, you should avoid yeast foods.

Beverages: Wine, saki, beer, all types of liquor, soda pop, any drinks flavored with artificial sweeteners, and all caffeine-containing drinks. Avoid all carbonated beverages during the eight-week program.

Foods You Can Eat

You can still eat hearty and tasty foods while on the candida overgrowth program. These include beef, lamb, poultry, eggs, fish, fresh vegetables by the pound, butter, and all the low-fat acidophilus culture yoghurt you want. The following list of foods you can enjoy while on the anti-candida diet is taken from the *Candida Cook Book*. Organic meats and vegetables are usually only found in health food stores.

Meats: Select fresh lean meats, poultry, and fish. Avoid ground meat, pork, breaded and pickled meats, or any processed meat. Try to buy only organic meat from animals fed no antibiotics, stimulants, or growth hormones. You can purchase organic beef from Coleman's Beef, 707 E. 50th, Denver, CO 80216 or ask your local health food store.

Dairy Products: Select fresh organic eggs, unsalted raw butter, low-fat milk, and low-fat acidophilus culture yogurt. (Fermented dairy products are NOT allowed, such as cheese, sour cream, buttermilk, etc.)

Seeds, Nuts, Legumes, and Grains: You may eat almonds, sunflower seeds, pumpkin seeds, and Brazil nuts, but no other kind of seeds or nuts. Be sure to use brown rice and whole grains. Puffed or crispy rice cakes are a good snack and go well with many foods. Keep carbohydrates at a minimum, about 60-80 grams a day, and try to select grains that have negligible gluten content. (High gluten grains include wheat, oats, rye, and barley.) You may have corn, buckwheat, millet, rice, and potatoes as your starch, but don't go overboard because carbohydrates in all forms feed candida when it is overgrown.

Yeast Products: All nutritional yeast products are allowed, including brewer's yeast, vitamins, flour, bread, and pasta. (Be sure there is no honey or sugar in the bread.) If you have a prior history of yeast sensitivity, you may wish to restrict yeast intake.

Produce: Select vegetables that look fresh and free of mold. Pass up the fruit section; however, lemons are acceptable.

Condiments: Select olive oil, spices, herbs, and sea salt. Read the spice labels carefully to be sure no yeast is present in spice blends.

Canned Goods: A few canned goods, without additives, such as tomato paste, water chestnuts, tuna, and sardines are acceptable for emergencies. Choose canned tomato products without citric acid.

Frozen Vegetables: Stock some, such as frozen artichoke hearts or green peas for soups and salads. Check labels for products containing sugar, vinegar, and additives.

Colon Therapy

You should have one colon cleansing each week or as needed. Bring one quart Pau D'Arco tea with you for your colon cleansing. This will help to relieve candida die-off symptoms.

Candida Die-off Reactions

During the eight-week program, it is not uncommon to experience some or many of the following symptoms, which can be attributed to the die-off reaction of the candida. These symptoms include feeling tired, spacey, dizzy, apathetic; or you may experience nausea, flulike symptoms, or a goopy sick feeling; muscular aches and pains, skin rashes, headaches, abdominal bloating, rectal itching, irritability, depression, food cravings, and difficulty in sleeping.

You can relieve some of these symptoms by getting plenty of rest at night, exercising, drinking at least eight glasses of water daily, eating regularly, and keeping snacks available throughout the day. Eating extra protein can also help relieve fatigue.

If you feel overly ill, you should stop the Caprystatin, Kaprycidin-A, and Orithrush-D Gargle (but continue with the other products) until you feel better—usually one or two days. Then continue with the program where you left off. This would mean that your program would be longer than eight weeks.

First Week

_____ Date Started _____Date Completed

Upon arising and just before bed, take DDS-1 and Travacid X. (Keep DDS-1 Acidophilus in the refrigerator.) Take the other products before meals.

DDS-1 Acidophilus   2 upon arising with water only and 2 before bedtime with water only

Travacid X	1 with DDS-1 upon arising and 1 before bedtime with water only

(Take the above two products at the same time.)

Caprystatin	1 twice daily before meals
Arizona Natural Garlic	2 twice daily before meals
Co-enzyme Q10	1 twice daily before meals
Intestinal Cleanser	2 twice daily before meals
Megavital	1 twice daily before meals

(Take the above five products at the same time.)

Pau D'Arco Tea	1 cup daily
	Directions: Add 1 heaping Tbs. Pau D'Arco Tea to 4 cups boiling water. Simmer 20 minutes. Strain and refrigerate. Drink either hot or cold.

Second Week

_____ Date Started _____ Date Completed

Take all products as in the first week, except increase Caprystatin as follows:

Caprystatin	2 twice daily before meals

Third Week

_____ Date Started _____ Date Completed

Take all products as in the first week, except increase Caprystatin as follows:

Caprystatin	3 twice daily before meals

Fourth Week

_____ Date Started _____ Date Completed

Take all products as in the first week with the exception of Caprystatin. Continue to take 3 Caprystatin twice daily through the eighth week. Begin Kaprycidin-A as follows:

Caprystatin	3 twice daily before meals
Kaprycidin-A	1 twice daily before meals

Fifth Week

_____ Date Started _____ Date Completed

Take all products as in the first week with the exception of Caprystatin and Kaprycidin-A. Continue to take 3 Caprystatin twice daily through the eighth week. Take Kaprycidin-A as follows:

Caprystatin	3 twice daily before meals
Kaprycidin-A	2 twice daily before meals

Sixth Week

_____ Date Started _____ Date Completed

Take all products as in the first week with the exception of Caprystatin and Kaprycidin-A. Continue to take 3 Caprystatin twice daily through the eighth week. Take Kaprycidin-A as follows:

Caprystatin	3 twice daily before meals
Kaprycidin-A	3 twice daily before meals

Seventh Week

_____ Date Started _____ Date Completed

Take all products as in the first week, with the exception of Caprystatin and Kaprycidin-A. Continue to take 3 Caprystatin and 3 Kaprycidin-A. Begin Orithrush-D Gargle as follows:

Caprystatin	3 twice daily before meals
Kaprycidin-A	3 twice daily before meals
Orithrush-D Gargle	Mix 1 part Orithrush with 20 parts water (no refrigeration

necessary); gargle and then swallow one mouthful of this mixture twice daily.

Eighth Week

_____ Date Started _____ Date Completed

Take all products as in the seventh week.

CONGRATULATIONS! You have completed the Candida Overgrowth Elimination Program! Now, you should continue with the following instructions.

---

1. After completing the eight-week program, discontinue the following products: Caprystatin, Kaprycidin-A, and Orithrush-D Gargle.

2. You will have some other products remaining after the eighth week. Finish the remainder of the following products as follows:

Intestinal Cleanser	2 twice daily before meals
Arizona Natural Garlic	2 twice daily before meals

3. Continue to take the following products for three months as follows:

DDS-1 Acidophilus	2 upon arising with water only and 2 before bedtime with water only
Travacid X	1 with DDS-1 upon arising and 1 before bedtime with water only

   (Take the above two products at the same time)

Co-enzyme Q10	1 twice daily before meals
Megavital	1 twice daily before meals

   (Take the above two products at the same time)

Pau D'Arco Tea	1 cup daily

4. Slowly add restricted foods back into your diet. For the first few days, only add fermented foods. For the next few days add sweet foods, such as fruits, juices, and honey. Try to avoid alcoholic beverages for 30 days.

   If you experience a recurrence of symptoms, return to the restricted diet for 30 days and take three Caprystatin twice daily before meals in addition to the products in instruction 3 above.

5. Avoid commercial meats, chicken, and eggs since they contain antibiotics, stimulants, growth hormones, and pesticides. Your local health food store should have organic meat, chicken (such as Rocky Road chicken), and eggs that are free of these chemicals. Choose wisely, ask questions, and don't settle for less than clean chemical-free food.

6. At some future time, due to illness, you may be required to take an antibiotic. After you have completed the full cycle of the medication, take two DDS-1 Acidophilus capsules twice daily to rebuild your intestinal flora. This will help you avoid any future candida overgrowth.

CHAPTER 7

Parasites: A Deadly Enemy

The first major nationwide survey of parasitic diseases has revealed that one in every six people studied has one or more parasites living somewhere in his body.

—Ronald Kotulak

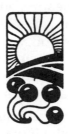

Parasites and Disease

Billions of people are afflicted with intestinal parasites or worms. These vermin cause greater susceptibility to disease and may cause weight problems as well. According to Dr. John Black, statistics show that in certain areas of the world more than 80 percent of the population has parasites. In North America alone, at least 21 million persons are afflicted. (Reported in Medical Encyl. Vol. 3, 1976, ed. Robert E. Rothenberg, M.D., F.A.C.S.).

The invasion of parasites, plus a clogged colon, can be the two main causes for many diseases, according to a panel of 75 eminent physicians at the Royal Society of Medicine in Great Britain.

Worms, such as pinworms, hookworms, ringworms, roundworms, and tapeworms, enjoy the undigested food residue that ends up plastered on the inside of the intestinal walls. Placque-filled intestine walls block the natural absorption of nutrients into the bloodstream, thus interrupting digestion. Dr. Henry Bieler says, "The first line of defense against disease is digestion."

Parasites feed upon this encrusted waste and grow fat and sassy, multiplying by the thousands. As many as seven varieties have been found present at one time in the colon. These worms vary in length from a fraction of an inch to over 30 feet.

Pinworms feed primarily on sweets and all refined carbohydrates that literally plate intestinal walls. Pinworms reside in the cecum, appendix, and colon (large intestine). Hookworms, usually from animal feces, attach themselves to the colon wall and feed off your blood. Ringworms and roundworms are also contracted from animal feces. Tapeworms are derived from improperly cooked meats, including pork, beef, fish, and also from animal feces.

People can also get worms from contact with pets, shaking hands with people who have pets, going barefoot, and even from eating raw fruits and vegetables that are infested with parasite eggs.

Worms Outrank Cancer
as Man's Deadliest Enemy

by Dolly Katz

Every year, the American Cancer Society publishes the names of famous people, such as Duke Ellington and Jack Benny, who have died of cancer. This is done, the society says, as "a dramatic reminder of the full dimensions of cancer's human devastation."

When Abdel Halim Hafez, the most popular singer in the Arab world, died last year, his name did not appear on any list, although the disease that killed him causes more human devastation than cancer does. Hafez, 46, died from complications of schistosomiasis, an infection of parasitic worms that live in the intestines. Worldwide, an estimated 200 million people—the equivalent of the entire U.S. population—are infected with this disease.

And the schistosomiasis worm is only one of many parasites, ranging in size from microscopic single-celled animals to foot-long roundworms, which annually kill many more people than cancer does. The diseases they cause are as well known as malaria and as obscure as kala-azar, which particularly affects children and is 90 percent fatal if untreated.

One of every four people in the world is infected by roundworms, which cause fever, cough, and intestinal problems. A quarter of the world's people have hookworms, which can cause anemia and abdominal pain. A third of a billion people suffer from the abdominal pain and diarrhea caused by whipworms.

Not much research is being done on these diseases. The U.S. spends more than $800 million a year on cancer research. All the nations of the world combined spend less than one-twentieth that amount studying parasitic diseases. As a result, there are no vaccines against them, and many of them are difficult or impossible to treat. There is no known treatment, for instance, for Chagas' disease, a variant of African sleeping sickness that occurs in South and Central America.

But while these diseases occur predominately in underdeveloped countries, the U.S. is not immune to them. Just about every parasitic disease known has been diagnosed in the U.S. in the last few years: schistosomiasis, trichinosis, giardiasis, toxoplasmosis, African sleeping sickness.

Most, like malaria, are imported cases brought back by travelers. But a significant number are entrenched in parts of our environment, kept alive in the U.S. by person-to-person transmission.

Pinworms, for example, parasites that live in the lower intestine and rectum, are the most common parasitic infection of children in temperate countries. At least one in five children in the general population has pinworms; in institutions, the figure can go as high as 90 percent.

All this doesn't mean that Americans ought to add parasites to the long list of diseases we're supposed to worry about when we develop symptoms. But it's interesting and perhaps important to realize that to most of the world's people, cancer is as exotic a disease as sleeping sickness is to us.

Reprinted from The Miami Herald, *June 25, 1978.*

Parasites More Common
than Believed, Study Says

by Ronald Kotulak

The first major nationwide survey of parasitic diseases has revealed that one in every six people studied has one or more parasites living somewhere in his body.

The prevalence of these parasitic stowaways, which range from microscopic organisms to 15-foot tapeworms, has come as a big surprise, especially to physicians who receive little training in diagnosing and treating parasitic infections.

"We think of this country as a highly sanitized country," Dr. Myron G. Schulz said, "but that is not necessarily true."

The large number of parasites, he said, means they are causing many diseases that baffle doctors.

"Many patients have experienced weeks of delay before the correct diagnosis was made and have been subjected to unnecessary laboratory tests, hospitalization, and even surgery," Shultz, director of the parasitic diseases division of the Centers for Disease Control (CDC) in Atlanta, warned in an editorial appearing in an upcoming issue of the *Journal of the American Medical Association*.

He said that the presence of parasites also means that many Americans are not as "clean" as they thought they were.

"What concerns me is that somewhere along the line there has been a breakdown in sanitation measures and people have ingested contaminated food, water, or dirt," said Dr. Dennis Juranek, assistant chief of the CDC's parasitic diseases division.

The survey pinpointed four problems:

- A parasite that causes intestinal infections is sweeping across the country. Called Giardia Lamblia, the parasite has now become the number one cause of waterborne disease in the nation.

- Tapeworm infections appear to have increased by 100 percent in the last ten years, an increase that may be linked to American's increasing fondness for raw or rare beef.

- Amebiasis, the most deadly of the parasites, continues to be a serious problem, with recent outbreaks in South Carolina. Between 1969 and 1973 there were 242 reported deaths from amebiasis, a microscopic organism usually passed from person to person.

- Illinois farmers are being plagued by a Balatidium parasite from pigs that causes intestinal infections in humans.

The survey involved examinations of 414,820 samples of feces in 1976. The examinations were performed by 570 public and private laboratories in all 50 states and the results sent to the CDC.

According to the survey, 15.6 percent of the specimens contained one or more parasites. About half these parasites are capable of causing disease.

The large number of parasitic infections discovered in the survey may not reflect the actual rate of infection in the general public, but it does reveal that the problem is much more widespread than most health professionals thought.

"I'm sure that this high infection rate comes as a surprise to those who never considered parasitic diseases to be a major problem in the U.S.," Dr. Juranek said.

The biggest problem uncovered in the survey was the high rate of infection with the Giardia parasite.

This parasite now appears to have spread to almost every state and is responsible for recent epidemics in upstate New York, Colorado, Washington, and New Hampshire.

This bug, a protozoan parasite, is microscopic in size and resembles a single-celled amoeba. The parasite coats the inside lining of the small intestine and prevents the lining from absorbing nutrients from food.

Although not a killer, it causes illness characterized by diarrhea, weakness, weight loss, abdominal cramps, nausea, vomiting, belching, and fever.

Most cases are misdiagnosed as bacterial infections, but unfortunately antibiotics have no effect on the parasite, Dr. Juranek said. Two drugs are effective in curing Giardias: atabrine, an antimalarial agent, and metronidazole.

Hundreds of small water systems throughout the country that do not adequately purify water may be contaminated with the parasite, said Dr. John Hoff, an EPA research microbiologist.

Streams or watersheds may become contaminated through infected human sewage, and recent studies show that Giardia-infected beavers may also contaminate water sources.

Reprinted from the Chicago Tribune Service.

Parasites and AIDS

by Rev. Hanna Kroeger

AIDS (Acquired Immune Deficiency Syndrome) is not one disease in itself. Rather it is caused by the accumulation of several factors that weaken the immune system so drastically that the body is susceptible to many other diseases.

Parasites, such as hookworm and protozoa, are found in almost all carriers of AIDS. The most common type of hookworm found, Hydatoxi Lualba, is microscopic and can travel into the lung tissue making lesions. It also can be found in the brain, intestines, rectum, and intracutaneous tissue. It is the same microscopic disturbance that causes uremic poisoning during pregnancy.

Widespread protozoa, a freshwater parasite causing weakening of the entire system, is also found in AIDS carriers. Protozoa do not suck blood as the hookworm does, but that make arthritislike pains, leukemia symptoms, bleeding under the skin, and a host of other symptoms. Dr. Bingham, author of the book *Fight Back Against Arthritis*, states on page 52:

> *Overall, it seems highly probable that various species of free-living protozoa are the etiological agent of collagene-anti-immune disease which show every graduation and combination with one another. They are not due to a single organism, but to a number of similar organisms. Such a parasitic infection would explain the urticaria asthma and easinophilia observed in many cases of collagene or auto-immune diseases.*

Sometimes flukes and flatworms are found in the blood of AIDS sufferers. These bloodflukes make lesions in the lungs and hemorrhages under the skin.

Finally, *Candida albicans*, the hidden epidemic, is *always* found in AIDS victims. This fungus overgrowth can affect every organ and part of the body and is the worst of the fungi that attack the nervous system.

Reprinted by permission of Rev. Hanna Kroeger, 7075 Valmont Drive, Boulder, CO 80301.

Parasites and Disease:
A Survival of the Fittest

by June M. Wiles, Ph.D.

The smaller the world becomes, the more susceptible we are to parasitic-induced diseases. With the present easy mode of travel between this country and foreign lands, new and unrecognized strains of parasites are being introduced that further challenge us to live defensively.

In the U.S. there are 500 known types of parasites: 200 types of friendly, microscopic creatures that actually help keep us alive and healthy or are not a threat to us; and 300 types ranging in size from microscopic to 25 feet long that can be our mortal enemies. Probably the largest known parasite at present, and the most troublesome in America, is the tapeworm.

Around the turn of the century, before hygiene reached its comfortable reassuring status, the family doctor and, in fact, every mother watched for worms and gave home remedies, such as several drops of kerosene in a spoonfull of sugar at least once per year. (I remember receiving this remedy and I am still amazed that I survived what I consider to be a very questionable treatment.)

Ecological balance from the beginning of time was and still is essential to our survival. Every plant and animal, right down to the smallest germ, plays an important role in man's survival. The basic premise of ecological balance is that the stronger creature lives off the weaker. But none is bad; all have a purpose and meet nature's demands for ecological balance.

If an organism becomes weak, there is always something down the chain of living matter prepared to invade it—that is, recognize it as a suitable source of food—and thus, in natural sequence, decomposition occurs, preparing the organism to return to the earth, whether it be plant, animal or man. Even the putrefactive bacteria that attack the food particles in the colon causing gas, weakness, loss of energy, and sometimes nausea, are part of the wholistic balance of nature. It is necessary through intelligent reasoning by man to introduce into the intestinal flora a proper bacteria, *Lactobacillus acidophilus*, compatible with his chemistry and capable of helping to counteract putrefaction and to achieve ecological balance in the colon. The basic premise is that unless we find a way to keep the colon clean and free of debris and parasites, we prematurely become part of the purging process of nature.

Excerpts from the book *RBTI Diet and Guidebook*, page 43, provide a more specific understanding of the problem:

Parasites are vermin that steal your food, drink your blood and leave their excrement in your body to be reabsorbed back into the bloodstream as nourishment.

There are approximately 25 varieties of parasites which *can be seen with the naked eye*. Some of these are pinworms, hookworms, roundworms, tapeworms and ringworms.

Many of these, most notably pinworms, feed primarily on sweets and refined sugars. They will develop colonies in the colon and rectum and leave the colon irritated and raw.

Hookworms, usually contracted from the fecal matter of animals, will attach themselves to the colon wall and suck blood from the feeder mouths of the villi in the colon that should transmit nourishment from the food we eat to our bloodstream. This worm is very prevalent in the South. It is conservatively estimated that 225,000,000 persons in the world allow this "freeloader" to drain their lives away. Hookworms cause anemia, abdominal pain, diarrhea, apathy, malnutrition, and even underdevelopment in children.

The ringworm is common and is contracted from animals. Direct application of Walnut Tincture on ringworm-infested areas will rid the body of this pest.

Tapeworms are derived from uncooked or poorly cooked meats. They feed on their host in the intestines or in muscle tissue.

Parents should stress to children the importance of washing hands after handling pets. Don't let animals lick hands and face and open sores. Keep pets off the furniture as eggs are deposited there. Use separate dishes and sterilize well. Clean sleep areas often. Keep sandals on children's feet. Do not allow them to go barefoot except in such places as the beach or protected playyard or sandbox.

Wash all salad stuffs in soda water (1 Tbs. to a quart of water) to remove parasite eggs.

Tapeworm eggs can also penetrate the membranes (feeder mouths intersticed in the villi) and travel to the liver where they set up housekeeping and suck nourishment from the liver. The fecal matter from a single tapeworm can make humans ill. The worms may become so numerous as to cause intestinal obstruction as well as gas and intestinal stress.

Tapeworm eggs in the liver are often mistaken for cancer and chemotherapy is administered. This mistaken diagnosis and treatment will kill the hydatid cyst (eggs) so they stop growing but may also kill the patient. The liver becomes too weak to discard the eggs, which slowly release toxins into the liver over a long period of time.

I know this situation occurred, because I did a lab study and isolated the eggs in the liver. The hospital and doctor were never sure the patient had cancer but "chemoed" his liver anyway, "just in case." Today this man is a walking dead man with a grossly swollen liver projected out front.

Tapeworms and other parasites can be destroyed harmlessly without injury to the body, by ingesting an intestinal cleanser called 6-N-1 along with the colon complements.

These colon complements are K-Min, castor oil capsules, and walnut tincture, which will kill almost every parasite known to man. Walnut tincture and K-Min can also be given to animals to rid them of parasites.

What is the secret of 6-N-1 Intestinal Cleanser?

- Every ingredient in 6-N-1 cleanser is natural and each serves a very specific purpose.
- The pH value is compatible with human chemistry.
- 6-N-1 is a superior roughage bulker.
- 6-N-1 carries the negative charge that is so essential to pull fecal impaction out of the pockets and crevices of a sick colon and into the gelatinous mass of 6-N-1 cleanser for expulsion from the body.
- 6-N-1 is the only colon cleanser on the market that is registered and trademarked!

Ingredients in 6-N-1 Intestinal Cleanser

Bentonite. Bentonite, a totally natural product of Mother Earth, is microscopic in size and carries a large and varied mineral content. This particular strain of bentonite is unequaled in controlling conditions of diarrhea where virus infections, food allergies, spastic colitis, and food poisoning exist. "Bentonite carries a strong negative electron and picks up 12 times its weight in positively charged toxic material from the colon wall for expulsion. The action of bentonite is purely physical and not chemical. Bentonite is used as a treatment in intestinal fermentation (gas), putrefaction, and harmful bacteria as well as parasites." (*Medical Annuals of Washington*, D.C., Vol. 20 (6), June 1961, The Value of Bentonite.)

Wheat Grass. Dr. Birscher, research scientist, calls wheat grass chlorophyl "concentrated Sun Power". Wheat grass also carries a negative electron and picks up eight times its weight in positively charged toxic material from the intestinal walls for expulsion. Wheat grass is known to increase the function of the heart, vascular system, intestines, uterus, and lungs. The wheat grass chlorophyll "raises the basic nitrogen exchange and is therefore a tonic without comparison." The gentle roughage of wheat grass releases clinging debris from intricate crevices of the bowel.

Whole Apple Fiber. Delicious Canadian apples, free of chemicals, make up whole apple fiber, which is loaded with vitamins, minerals, protein, and life -saving pectin and lipids. It also provides a gentle "brushing" and cleansing of the intestinal wall. The apple seeds provide nitrilosides.

Citrus Pectin and Plantago Avato. These capture putrefactive bacteria for expulsion. The jelling effect of pectin and plantago avato make them especially advantageous in this formula. The two are invaluable in forming a gentle colloidal mass for capturing and holding in suspension the impacted toxic material pulled from the walls of the colon. Citrus pectin is known for releasing heavy metals, such as mercury and lead, from the cells for expulsion. Citrus pectin is reported to help counteract the effects of radiation, cut cholesterol in blood, and reduce risk of heart attacks.

Herbs. Nature's natural medicines are part of the plan for man's survival. 6-N-1 Intestinal Cleanser contains gentian, golden seal, buckthorn, rhubarb root, cascara sagrada, and freeze-dried aloe vera, all well-calculated and delicately balanced in proportions essential for the success of the cleanser and detoxifier. This grouping pulls mucous, detoxifies, heals, acts as a diuretic, activates flushing of the liver and production of bile, and improves intestinal peristalsis.

Lactobacillus Acidophilus. Acidophilus is essential for balancing body chemistry. The purpose of acidophilus in this formula is to reinforce the production of healthy bacteria in the colon. Where there is too little acidophilus, gas forms, stools become putrid, and the normal production of Vitamin K is destroyed. When Vitamin K is destroyed, internal hemorrhaging can occur. When folic acid becomes deficient, the body cannot manufacture enough maintenance B complex to stabilize the nerves, and thus energy levels diminish and halitosis tells the sordid story.

Intestinal bacteria make up 80 percent of the stool and must be kept healthy to prevent growth of histamine. Histamine causes allergies and liberation of too much ammonia, which irritates delicate intestinal membrane and passes into the blood, causing nausea, vomiting, and gross toxicity. Putrefactive bacteria cause excessive growth of monilia albacans in the vaginal tract, leading to yeast infection. This infection can and does frequently spread to the lungs.

Bowel movements should be normal but larger than usual. By drinking approximately one half your body weight in ounces of water per day, you will maintain the moisture balance in the colon and assist flushing of waste material.

Colon Complements

The colon complements are an important part of the 6-N-1 program for good health. The addition of castor oil, K-Min, and walnut tincture is a superior way of stabilizing and balancing the chemical makeup of the colon.

K-Min. K-Min is a combination product of elements gathered above the earth and mined from the earth. K-Min will, by ionization, take worms apart; rarely will parasites pass out of the body whole. K-Min is a very effective compound in removing parasites from the colon. When the colon is free of parasites, yeast infection will usually clear up. The combination of K-Min and walnut tincture is effective against fungi, skin infections (due to microscopic parasites), ringworms, and larvae from the large intestines.

Walnut Tincture. In choosing an herb, it was necessary to choose one that would fight parasites throughout the body. The selection of walnut tincture was promoted by claims and experiences so grandiose I almost feel as if I must erect a shrine to the lowly walnut hull. It is not easily gathered, nor is the development of walnut tincture a simple process, but every step beginning to end is worth it. Needless to say, I look upon it with awe.

Walnut tincture is an excellent source of manganese. When tension is present in the intestinal tract, walnut tincture is a tremendously soothing healant. The elements in walnut tincture are unsurpassed for helping to strengthen ligaments, tendons, and muscles. The book, *Indian Herbology of North America*, states that black walnut tincture will assist in the healing of acne, burning in the anus, pain over the eyes, gas, headaches, herpes, scurvy, and pain in spleen, as well as syphillus, ulcers, rickets, and TB.

Castor Oil Capsules: Castor oil, when encapsulated and frozen, will go through the stomach and small bowel before opening. By freezing castor oil, the traditional cramping is totally eliminated because the capsules dissolve in the small intestine and specifically in the ileum (the last three fifths of the small intestine). It is here that the digestive tract hydrolizes this oil into recinoleic acid, which is harmless to humans but deadly to parasites.

The ileum connects to the cecum by way of the ileocecal valve. The majority of parasites of all kinds will nest in the cecum area (the lower end of the ascending colon where the large bowel begins). This area is warm and moist, providing a plentiful source of fresh food for these poisonous invaders.

Castor oil not only suffocates parasites, but is nature's penetrating oil for colon plaque. When the castor oil capsule is FROZEN it does not act as a laxative. Castor oil is odorless and will not "burp" back.

DDS-1 Acidophilus: Although the 6-N-1 Cleanser contains some acidophilus culture, I highly recommend additional acidophilus during the program in the form of DDS-1. This is a most opportune time to rebuild and rebalance the intestinal flora. Take two DDS-1 capsules first thing in the morning with water only and then two capsules at bedtime with water only.

The Immune System and AIDS

Parasites are a serious threat to a strong immune system. If we do not protect ourselves, we become prime targets for the AIDS virus, which literally destroys the immune system. The National Academy of Science says even HIV (human immunodeficiency virus) in the blood means at least a 25 to 50 percent chance of manifesting AIDS within five to ten years of infection, and that estimate may be low.

We can defend ourselves and fight back now by keeping our bodies clean and free of harmful bacteria and parasites. 6-N-1 Intestinal Cleanser and the colon complements— K-Min, walnut tincture, castor oil capsules, and DDS-1 Acidophilus—taken regularly morning and night will destroy parasites, cleanse, and correct severe imbalance in the colon.

Reprinted by permission of June M. Wiles, Ph.D., L.M.T., R.C.T., Holistic Health Clinic, 5025 East Fowler Avenue #13, Tampa, FL 33617; (813) 988-7788.

Eight-Week Parasite Elimination Program for Adults

Products Needed to Complete the Eight-Week Program

- 6-N-1 Intestinal Cleanser

  (If you weigh under 100 lbs.—3 bottles. If you weigh 101–175 lbs.—3 bottles. If you weigh over 175 lbs.—4 bottles.)

- DDS-1 Acidophilus capsules—3 bottles
- K-Min—2 bottles
- Black Walnut Tincture—4 ounces
- Castor Oil Capsules:

  If you weigh under 100 lbs.—2 bottles

  If you weigh 101–175 lbs.—3 bottles

  If you weigh over 175 lbs. —4 bottles

The order form for these products is on page 188.

Directions and Special Instructions
- Take these products twice daily, immediately upon arising and 30 to 45 minutes before retiring. No dietary changes are required, although reduction of sugar is desirable.

- Castor oil capsules must be taken FROZEN. Put them in the freezer one or two days before you begin the program. Take frozen castor oil capsules ten minutes before 6-N-1 Intestinal Cleanser capsules.

- Mix black walnut tincture with six ounces of distilled water. Follow with K-Min capsules and another six to eight ounces of distilled water.

- Drink at least eight glasses of water daily to help flush toxins from the body.

- Enemas and colonics hasten expulsion of waste. Try to have a colonic once a week during the program to flush out parasites and other toxins.

Schedule for Adults

By Weight	6-N-1 Intestinal Cleanser	Frozen Castor Oil	K-Min	Black Walnut Tincture
Under 100 lbs.	4 caps. 2 x day	3 caps. 2 x day	3 caps. 2 x day	20 drops 2 X day
101– 175 lbs.	5 caps. 2 x day	4 caps. 2 x day	3 caps. 2 x day	25 drops (or 1/4 tsp.) 2 x day
Over 175 lbs.	6 caps. 2 x day	6 caps. 2 x day	3 caps. 2 x day	25 drops (or 1/4 tsp.) 2 x day

Regardless of weight, take two capsules of DDS-1 Acidophilus first thing in the morning with water only and then two capsules at bedtime with water only.

Four-Week Parasite Elimination Program for Children

Products Needed to Complete the Four-Week Program

- 6-N-1 Intestinal Cleanser—1 bottle
- DDS-1 Acidophilus—1 bottle
- K-Min—1 bottle
- Black Walnut Tincture—1 bottle
- Castor Oil—1 bottle

The order form for these products is on page 188.

Schedule for Children

Age	6-N-1 Intestinal Cleanser	Frozen Castor Oil	K-Min	Black Walnut Tincture
1–6	1 cap. 2 x day	1 cap. 2 x day	1/2 cap. 2 x day	10 drops 2 x day in 3 oz. water
6–13	2 caps. 2 x day	1 cap. 2 x day	1 cap. 2 x day	15 drops 2 x day in 3 oz. water
Over 13	Follow Adult Program			

Regardless of age, take one capsule of DDS-1 Acidophilus first thing in the morning with water only and then one capsule at bedtime with water only.

Directions and Special Instructions

- Have children take all products twice daily, immediately upon arising and 30 to 45 minutes before retiring. No dietary changes are necessary except to reduce intake of sugar products.

- Castor oil capsules must be taken FROZEN. Put them in the freezer one or two days before beginning the program. Have children take frozen castor oil capsules ten minutes before 6-N-1 Intestinal Cleanser capsules.

- Mix black walnut tincture with six ounces of distilled water. Follow with K-Min capsules and another six to eight ounces of distilled water.

- All products should be taken for four weeks; however, children aged one to six should only take K-Min for seven days.

- Water enemas are suggested once a week.

- Though it is difficult to get some children to drink water, measure out distilled water to equal one half of the child's weight in ounces and encourage the child to drink it throughout the day. Remember, water is one part oxygen—children need it!

- Although additional acidophilus culture is not required after completing the Parasite Elimination Program, this is a most opportune time to rebalance the intestinal flora. For this reason I would suggest children take two capsules of DDS-1 Acidophilus daily for an additional thirty days.

CHAPTER 8

Metabolic Typing: The Commonsense Guide to Proper Nutrition

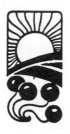

Metabolic Typing:
The Commonsense Guide
to Proper Nutrition

by William L. Wolcott

Many people have asked, "What do I need to do to achieve optimum health?" A large number of health-conscious individuals, failing to find proper guidance in the marketplace, discover for themselves that even by eating the very best organic foods and taking all the finest nutritional supplements money can buy, they still do not feel completely well. Moreover, what seems to work for some people, making them feel better or improving their adverse symptoms, in others has little or no effect, and in still others, actually appears to *worsen their health situation!*

If you (or anyone else for that matter) do not already know the answer to that question, finding out can prove to be an overwhelming undertaking. Little help of any real value can be gained from traditional medicine whose focus is on treating disease rather than on building health. A typical response from the average physician, when asked the above question, is to advise you to merely eat a well-balanced diet. But when you ask the next logical question, "What is a well-balanced diet for me?" you probably receive little, if any, meaningful information at all.

Creating Clarity from Confusion

Take heart, for there does appear to be a solution to all of this! Although we don't claim to have all the answers, HEALTHEXCEL has made an exciting and promising breakthrough by providing a framework for understanding what appears to be a hopeless morass of confusing and conflicting information about which foods to eat and which supplements to take in order to be healthy.

HEALTHEXCEL is an organization dedicated to the acceleration of the unfoldment of human potential through the creation of excellence in health. The basis for this unfoldment is a provocative, health-building program that is structured in an individualized approach to nutrition known as the HEALTHEXCEL System of Metabolic Typing.

You have probably heard it said, "You are what you eat." However, a much more accurate expression would be, "You are what you metabolize." Metabolism is the conversion of nutrients to energy, and the best way to know your unique nutritional needs is through an integrated approach of experimentation, observation, and the science of metabolic typing.

Metabolic typing is a highly complex procedure that requires the use of computer technology to analyze an enormous amount of personal data concerning each person's unique metabolic characteristics in order to determine individual nutritional requirements.

The concept of unique individual requirements for nutrition is certainly not an original idea brought forth by HEALTHEXCEL, nor even is the term "metabolic typing." The ancient Greek physicians, such as Hippocrates, recognized in their writings the validity of addressing the needs of the whole person, rather than just the symptoms of disease. To paraphrase their thinking on the subject, they recognized that different people had different kinds of maladies and that one man's food was another man's poison. Similar concepts can also be found in the ancient healing arts in the Far East, such as the yin and yang of Chinese medicine, and the correlation of the five elements to individual classifications in the Ayurvedic medicine of India.

Modern, progressive-minded researchers have revived this notion of health being dependent on our ability to obtain all the nutrients for which we have a genetic requirement. Dr. Roger Williams, the noted biochemist from the University of Texas, expounded his genetotrophic principle in which he showed that our individual characteristics, which are an expression of our uniqueness, are based in our genes and that these genetically inherited differences extend to even the level of the individual cell in determining the rate of individual cellular activity.

According to Dr. Williams, *all people are genetically predisposed to specific biochemical needs, which if not met, lead to degenerative disease*. This he termed a person's biochemical individuality. He believes that all degenerative disease, including cancer, is caused by such "cellular malnutrition."

Dr. Williams advocates the need ". . . to develop techniques for identifying the inherited pattern of susceptibilities and resistances that is unique to each individual. This metabolic profile represents a necessary precondition for making rational programs of nutrition, tailored to fit each individual's special requirements."

Other independent metabolic and nutritional researchers concurrently developed just such metabolic typing systems for the determination of individual nutritional requirements. Many researchers, such as Dr. Francis Pottenger and Dr. R. O. Muller, worked with individual classification through the autonomic nervous system. Dr. William Donald Kelley coined the term "metabolic typing" and was the first to utilize computer technology to analyze nutritional needs based on the autonomic nervous system. Dr. George Watson's research, and later that of Dr. Paul Eck, centered around the oxidation rate, the rate at which nutrients are burned for energy in the cells, as the basis for the determination of individual nutritional needs. Other researchers, such as Dr. Henry Bieler, Dr. Melvin Page, and Dr. Elliot Abravanel, developed means of classification through analysis of the endocrine system.

It has become quite clear that the acquisition of good health is dependent on good nutrition. It has also become quite clear that what is right for one person, as the ancient Greeks knew, is not necessarily correct for someone else. What constitutes good nutrition for the Eskimo is not the same as for the vegetarian East Indian. However, knowing your ancestry alone is not of much practical value, for it has become apparent that children from the same parents may not only differ to the extreme in external appearances and personalities, but also in terms of their nutritional requirements. This is particularly true of our modern society in America, which today is a genetic melting pot of the world.

However, the fact that your inherited nutritional requirements may be a matter of genetic roulette does not diminish the imperative need to meet those requirements. The bottom line still is that in order to be healthy, you *must* supply the body with all the raw materials, vitamins, minerals, and enzymes for which it has a genetic need. The failure to do so results in inefficiency of function of cells, organs, glands, and systems, imbalance in body chemistry, and eventually medically diagnosable dis-ease [sic].

Obviously, every vitamin and mineral is vital and necessary, but different people need *different amounts of the different nutrients.* Amazing as it may seem, it is very likely that most of the books touting the various nutrients are correct. *However, the books are accurate only for certain specific metabolic types; their recommendations are incorrect for other metabolic types!* This is what has made the field of nutrition so confusing.

What is an even more remarkable discovery now expounded by HEALTHEXCEL is that not only do different people need different amounts of nutrients, but also *any given nutrient can have an opposite reaction in different people. This explains why what improves one person's condition can actually worsen the same condition in someone else.* This discovery—that the way any given nutrient affects an individual depends upon the metabolic type of that individual—must be taken into account or any research experiments regarding the effects of nutrients will be quite meaningless.

This important understanding has yet another implication: *Any given health problem cannot be successfully addressed by a symptom-treatment approach.* To illustrate, consider the common problem of leg cramps. Leg cramps usually are an indication of a disruption of calcium metabolism. The common solution is to take additional calcium, and indeed for some metabolic types this is an effective and proper solution. But, few people realize that in other metabolic types this course of action provides not a solution but rather a worsening of the problem. For these metabolic types what is needed is not the ingestion of more calcium, but rather a diminishment of dietary calcium and an increase of those nutrients that are the biochemical "opposite," such as potassium and magnesium, in order to improve the utilization of calcium.

The principle illustrated with this relatively simple health adversity holds true for most all health problems as well. In order to successfully deal with an adverse health situation, it is imperative that you first understand the metabolic type in question before any recommendations are made. Only in this way can you be assured of getting your "medicine" and not your "poison." *The answer to the question regarding proper nutrition for any individual can only be obtained once the metabolic type of the individual is understood.*

The HEALTHEXCEL System

Through the HEALTHEXCEL System of Metabolic Typing, the clouds of confusion may be dispelled by providing a scientific (i.e., systematic, testable, repeatable, and verifiable) answer to the question regarding what you can do in order to be healthy. More than seven years of empirical research into the relationship of metabolic typing to the determination of individual nutritional requirements has uncovered a common denominator to all the systems of metabolic evaluation: energy! This realization has led to the further discovery that the previous systems of evaluation developed by the pioneers of metabolic nutritional research are in themselves neither right nor wrong, but are instead pieces of the same puzzle that complement rather than oppose each other.

Genes dictate the characteristics of each individual cell—the structure and purpose of the cell, the rate of cellular activity, the nutrients required by the cell for repairing and rebuilding, for reproduction, for energy production, and for successful completion of all cellular activities. Cells group together based upon similar makeup and purpose to form organs, glands, and other bodily tissues. These, in turn, form the various systems in the body whose purposes are to perform the special functions of the digestive system, the immune system, and so forth.

Metabolic Typing: Understanding Body Language

The HEALTHEXCEL System of Metabolic Typing is a process of evaluation of the interrelationship of the body's three main systems for the creation, maintenance, and control of energy: the autonomic nervous system, the oxidative system, and the endocrine system.

The nutrients obtained by the body from air, food, water, and light provide the fuel for all the processes of metabolism. By supplying the body with all the raw materials for which it has a genetic requirement, you set the stage for optimum energy production, the essential ingredient for good health and well-being.

Every activity in the body, whether it be physiological, psychological or biochemical in nature, depends on the rate, quality, and amount of energy available. When the mind is clear and sharp, there is ample energy for emotional experience, and physical energy abounds. All the body's cells, organs, glands, and systems function efficiently and harmoniously. An overall feeling of vitality and well-being naturally pervades your experience.

But when the cells are deficient in their fuel requirements, and metabolic activity becomes disrupted, imbalanced and inefficient, then the quality of your experience on all levels reflects that condition. The body then begins to communicate in its own "language" the fact that all is not well!

At first, it might just appear as a lessening of energy, of mental sharpness or of emotional interest. Then actual non-specific symptoms or conditions, which are undiagnosable as an actual disease process, may begin to appear—such as headaches, digestive disturbances, constipation, food sensitivities; emotional disruptions, such as anger, irritability, depression for no apparent reason; apathy, lethargy, loss of interest in life, weight problems, loss of sex drive, disruption of energy levels, and so forth. If not corrected, such biochemical deficiencies may eventually give way to a full-blown diagnosable degenerative disease.

But, long before that time, the body will have been communicating in its own fashion the fact that all is not well. The interpretation and the understanding of this body language is the quest of metabolic typing. In its own way, the body constantly defines its individuality; it gives expression to its imbalances and makes known the need for its requirements. The mental, emotional, and physical characteristics the body displays supply an ample description and unending flow of information regarding its status quo. You need only develop an understanding of the principles involved in metabolic typing in order to begin to understand the language of the body.

This understanding is effectively accomplished through HEALTHEXCEL's H.O.P.E. Survey (Health Optimization Profile Evaluation): a 1,000-question computerized analysis that seeks an understanding of the physiological basis for the numerous and varied characteristics that comprise your individual metabolic experience. Understanding the physiological basis for all your characteristics allows for a categorization of all the known characteristics. Then, overall metabolic patterns and styles of functioning may be seen and the metabolic classification may be determined, based upon the three main energy systems of the body: the autonomic, oxidative, and endocrine systems. Once this is accomplished, nutritional recommendations in terms of diet and supplementation appropriate for your unique metabolic requirements can be made.

Then, by eating the very best organic foods *that are correct for your metabolic type*, by taking nutritional supplements *that are suitable for your nutritional individuality*, by avoiding toxins in your food and in your environment, by having regular structural treatments, and by cleansing and detoxifying your body regularly, you can truly make headway on the road to your optimal health and well-being!

Information about HEALTHEXCEL

HEALTHEXCEL, Inc., based in the foothills of the North Cascades in Eastern Washington State, is an education and information service company. Working through an established and growing referral network of health professionals, including medical doctors, dentists, osteopaths, chiropractors, nutritional consultants, and other health-related professionals, HEALTHEXCEL provides important information concerning individual nutritional requirements gleaned from complex and comprehensive computerized evaluation procedures.

Professionals employing the HEALTHEXCEL program in their practice can receive additional information and guidance by telephone from 10:00 a.m. to 10:00 p.m., Pacific time. Discussions center around the 100-page reports provided by HEALTHEXCEL as a result of the evaluation procedure, which includes valuable information about individual nutritional requirements. Extensive information is provided concerning each person's metabolic type, supplement recommendations, which foods are most appropriate for the individual's metabolism as well as why those foods are recommended and how they will effect one's metabolism.

If you decide that you would like to know more about metabolic typing or what it would entail to find out about your unique nutritional requirements, you are invited to call or write to HEALTHEXCEL at the following address: HEALTHEXCEL, Inc., Route 1, Box 495, Winthrop, WA 98862; (509) 996-2131.

Printed by permission of William L. Wolcott.

CHAPTER 9

Articles by Other Authors

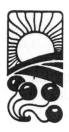

High-Colonic Irrigation

by Carol Signorella

*Suppose you've jogged, dieted, gulped your vitamins, yet still feel
fagged out and frail. This writer despaired of ever being jazzily
vital, until she rediscovered a decades-old method of releasing
natural energy. . .*

"Colonic what?" I exclaimed.

"Colonic irrigation," Connie explained. "Like an internal
bath to wash the poisons out of your system. You already
know about all the unwanted food additives in our diets, and
just think of the little extras not listed on the label. The
pesticides sprayed on your fruits and vegetables, the
hormones and antibiotics fed your beef and poultry. And
then, if you want to talk about pollution. . . ."

"All right, Connie. So what happens when you're irri-
gated?"

"Simplicity itself. Water—tap water, usually—is slowly
pumped up into the colon, our large intestine."

"An enema," I shuddered.

"In a way. But more water—an average of 25 to 30
gallons—is used and, under gentle pressure, it travels and
cleanses the length of your colon, washing out all the stale

bile and putrified waste poisoning your system. A colonic only takes an hour and is completely painless. You might even sleep through it."

Hmmmm, not likely, I thought. Still I had to admit that Connie's appearance had certainly improved since her first colonic irrigation three months before. Her eyes, skin, and hair all glowed. In fact, it's hard to describe Connie without making her sound like an ad for Short & Sassy.

That evening on the subway (where I do most of my serious thinking), I tallied my complaints: burning, itching eyes; yellow, dull skin; depression; anxiety; muddled head, uncoordinated body. Energy plummeted to a dreary low. For years I'd been busily trying out every possible cure for my persistent physical/emotional malaise; I'd jogged, quit smoking and drinking, added bran and dried fruit to my diet, even experimented with megavitamin therapy, but all to little avail. I remained dragged out, anxious, and definitely not my most vital self!

Why give up now? I thought. Maybe colonics could be a solution. Still, I wasn't going to let Connie talk me into anything without doing some independent research first. Naturally enough, I started with the American Medical Association—they, however, were less than helpful: "The AMA," I was told, "has no definitive statement on colonic irrigations; we neither recommend them nor are against them." A trip to the library at Columbia University College for Physicians and Surgeons proved equally unenlightening; their latest text on colonics was a 1927 volume titled *Troubles We Don't Talk About.*

The first professional opinion I sought also proved to be discouraging. My internist, Dr. Richard Nachtigall, who has a thriving Park Avenue practice, advised me to forget colonics. "I can't see much use for these irrigations," he said. "I've never heard of any real proof that they are useful except for certain abnormal conditions such as a defective liver, where it is necessary to remove bacteria-producing toxins." Dr. Milton Brothers, husband of Dr. Joyce Brothers, was even more emphatic: "I would never recommend them. It's an archaic practice and could be harmful. Colonics may induce a condition called electrolyte depletion. The bowel needs certain electrolytes—essential salts, acids, and alkalis—to perform its functions properly, and this sort of intensive irrigation could deplete the colon of these substances."

Not yet entirely deterred, I consulted another physician who believed colonics could improve health. "Nobody is really certain," he said, "where those all-important electrolytes are conserved, nor can any certain case be made for irrigation affecting their presence in the colon." Admitting that he personally believed in colonics (without including them in his practice), he also told me that these treatments are very popular among the rich and celebrated on the West Coast and in Europe. "Of course, it's just not something people want to talk about much," he explained, and then asked me to keep his name confidential. My anonymous source did, however, refer me to a Manhattan chiropractor and physical therapist who regularly performs this procedure, Dr. H. William Baum.

Dr. Baum, whose spritely step and taut, satinlike complexion belie his 85 years, practices naturopathic medicine; that is, he treats sickness primarily through natural means, believing that drugs and surgery should be resorted to only in extreme cases. Taking the holistic approach to health, the naturopath views disease not as an isolated malfunction, but rather as an indication that the entire body is in a state of "disease."

For over 60 years, Dr. Baum has been performing colonic irrigations and has never found them less than effective and safe. I mentioned the negative views of the physicians I'd consulted, but Dr. Baum remained unfazed. "Most doctors don't prescribe vitamins, either," he said, sensibly enough. Reassured by Dr. Baum's manner and remembering the glow colonics had brought to my friend Connie, I swallowed hard and asked to be treated.

The first step was familiar enough; I changed into a pair

of paper slippers and one of those thin, hospital-green gowns that open at the back. Then, clutching a pamphlet about colonics, I climbed aboard the long leather table and lay down on my side. The rectal applicator was inserted and the irrigation process began.

Throughout the colonic, I was attached to what resembled an old-fashioned water cooler, about four feet high and placed on the end of the examining table. When Dr. Baum pulled a lever in one direction, water burst into the clean, glass tank until it reached halfway to the top. Then the lever was reversed, and water began to slowly feed into me. The doctor moderated the pressure so that the water slowly worked its way through the twists and turns, obstructions and gases of the long large intestine.

After awhile, I realized with something like amazement that the water slushing up my intestinal tract had risen to just under my rib cage. Even so, I felt relaxed and experienced no pain. Dr. Baum's irrigation was much less unpleasant than either a home or hospital enema. I was not relaxed enough to drift right off to sleep, but I felt sufficiently comfortable to chat with Dr. Baum and learn a bit more about how and why colonics work . . . .

The indigestible portion of the food you eat, Dr. Baum explained, lodges in the large intestine and stays there until eliminated in a bowel movement. Infrequent movements or periods of constipation can, however, result in a partial decomposition of these waste substances that encrust the colon and further hinder elimination. These toxins are then reabsorbed into the bloodstream, lowering the body's defense against bacteria and viruses. The body strains to fight against the poisons and, if the effort is too great, various organs or even the circulatory system itself can break down. The early indications of this futile war against waste, Dr. Baum continued, include sallow skin, nervous irritability, coated tongue, bad breath, offensive body odor, headaches, bloating, poor appetite, and a feeling of stomach heaviness—symptoms that bore a marked resemblance to my own complaints.

Colonics might not be necessary, Dr. Baum went on, if Americans had enough bulk in their diets, exercised regularly, and avoided alcohol, tobacco, polluted air, and processed foods. Few of us, however, do lead such uncontaminated lives.

Why, I wondered, can some people smoke and drink and eat poorly and still remain in good physical health? Dr. Baum explained that this lucky group has a tremendous natural capacity to eliminate toxins from their systems; but even so, he advised me not to be too jealous. "Their bad habits will catch up with them someday."

Colonic irrigations can be performed with varying frequency. Dr. Baum thinks first-time patients should have three in a row to be sure they're thoroughly cleansed, and after that, the number of treatments "depends on what I see coming out of you." A few people have one a week for years, others one a month, while most people are satisfied with three or four irrigations a year, often timing their treatments to correspond with the change of seasons.

"The shift to warm or cold weather," says Dr. Baum, "can upset the body's rhythms. An irrigation helps you adjust. Actually, these treatments aren't designed to cure any specific ailment; rather, they're designed to tune up the system so it becomes more capable of healing itself."

I asked Dr. Baum if a laxative would be equally effective. His answer was an emphatic no: "Colonics involve only the large intestine," he explained, "while laxatives pass through the small intestine as well. That's where digestion and absorption of nutrients occur, vital processes that should not be interfered with. Besides, emetics are, in a sense, addictive— for them to continue to be effective, you need to take larger doses."

So, with irrigation, the small intestine is left to itself (as it should be) and only the toxins contained in the colon are washed away. Dr. Baum's reasoning seemed sound enough to me as my hour-long irrigation drew to a close and I prepared to reap the benefits of his ministrations.

As I climbed off the treatment table, I felt wonderful—high, energetic, positive, and strong. Before I left his office, Dr. Baum told me to take it easy the rest of the day and then suggested I change my diet to include lots of fresh fruits and vegetables, as well as plenty of bulk, and that I stay away from refined or processed foods. These changes would improve bowel functioning, he said, and lead to better overall health as well. I left feeling both peppy and inspired.

A few hours later, however, my high had completely faded, I was nauseous, dizzy, and nervously dialing Dr. Baum. He was not just reassuring, but positively congratulatory as I reeled off my symptoms. "That's the body continuing where the treatment left off," he told me. "The irrigation obviously stirred up a lot of poison. Eat something mild at regular intervals, rest, and come back in a few days for another treatment."

I did just that and continued the treatments once a month for nearly a year, sometimes adding an extra one when life was particularly stressful. I also followed Dr. Baum's advice about diet and within a few months noticed that I no longer had to discipline myself to eat properly. My craving for sugar had disappeared—I genuinely preferred an apple or helping of low-fat yogurt to a rich sweet. I also found myself developing a queasy aversion to coffee, cigarettes, and foods with preservatives—my body had learned to be naturally repelled by toxic substances.

After a year of colonics, my appearance and energy levels were both radically improved. No more draggy mornings or late-afternoon slumps. The bags under my eyes have disappeared entirely, and the sallow, yellowish tone that had spoiled my skin has been replaced by a healthy glow. I seem to think more clearly now, and I need less sleep. In a word, both my body and mind feel marvelously clean.

I couldn't be more enthusiastic about colonics.

Reprinted from Cosmopolitan Magazine.

Colonic Irrigation

by Angela Bell

The body comes into this world already knowing how to function in harmony—if its natural healing mechanisms are not interfered with. No one needs to teach a baby how to nurse or perform basic life processes of breathing, digestion, and elimination.

If the basic life processes somehow get out of balance, our inner environment can become a breeding ground for disease. Disease is not something that attacks us from without; it thrives in a mental and physical environment of lowered resistance that we allow.

If we neglect the body by feeding it improperly, failing to cleanse it inside or out, or treating it with disdain, we begin to create an inner environment where disease can flourish. The physical system then begins to rebel. In every way possible it tries to tell us to stop and evaluate our actions and thoughts—just as a true and loving friend might. Very often the body signals us with minor but annoying physical symptoms; these are not the disease, but only the outer signs of an imbalanced inner process.

Most of us never pay attention to these little warnings until we come down with a major dis-ease [sic]; then comes the mad race to eliminate symptoms (instead of the causes of disease). Unfortunately, this is not real healing. One of the warnings manifests as improper digestion and elimination.

Digestion is a multifaceted process. As food is taken into the mouth, the inner organs start a beautiful rhythmic dance. The esophagus moves rhythmically in a peristaltic action and moves the food into the stomach; the stomach begins its dance and then pushes the food into the small intestine. The small intestine begins its peristaltic movement, and thousands of tiny villi absorb the nutrients needed by the body and carry them into the bloodstream. (The villi also hold and later expel what the body does not need and cannot absorb.)

In a healthy person, the ileocecal valve opens and lets pass the waste that the small intestine has filtered out. Then, countless nerves are alerted to action, and this five and a half foot organ rhythmically begins to push waste from the lower right side of the abdomen upward past the liver. At this point, the intestine turns across to the spleen, where it turns again, and then travels down to the floor of the pelvis, where it empties.

This process should occur every time we eat. The person who does not eliminate after every meal is constipated. If this occurs, the body begins to reabsorb its own waste and this situation provides an environment where disease can flourish.

Over a period of time, if the colon loses its ability to have a regular, rhythmic peristaltic flow, its nerve signals stop functioning and large deposits of waste gradually lodge in its many pockets and convolutions. This waste paralyzes the ileocecal valve, backs up into the small intestine, and is reabsorbed into the bloodstream. Parasites as well as bacteria flourish in this environment. Once the colon's flexures (turns) are plugged, it cannot support peristaltic action; it loses its "memory" and no longer functions in a healthy way.

Several things may cause the colon to "freeze" and its contents to back up:

1. Emotional stress may cause a tightening of the solar plexus nerve centers, inhibiting proper breathing and thus the flow of energy into the colon.

2. Improper dietary habits: white flour, devitalized or preserved foods, too much meat, spices, sugar, milk products; certain food allergies, etc.

3. Mental stress, mostly subconscious; previous poor toilet training, negative attitudes or anxiety about one's body functions.

These problems can be remedied without dependence on habit-forming laxatives. One solution is colonics.

Colonic irrigation is a cleansing process that uses a special machine to introduce warm water to the entire colon. Colonics are a safe, rapid way of unplugging the body's sewage system when it is no longer working effectively.

Colonic irrigation cannot be compared to an enema; it functions in a different manner. Enemas only empty the lower 12 inches of the five and a half foot colon. The colonic irrigation reaches the entire length of the colon to the ileocecal valve; water flows out at the same rate it flows in. The process is painless, pleasant, and highly effective. It can remove the cause of chronic constipation and other diseases of the colon. The action of the water flowing in and being very gently drawn out through a very mild vacuum reminds the colon how to function on its own.

Once the colon regains its memory, it knows how to eliminate properly and no longer needs treatment. It does not need constant enemas to empty it; these tend to stretch and distort the lower rectal area of the colon and deaden the evacuation nerve impulses.

Once the colon is unblocked, self-maintenance is possible. We can keep our physical and mental channels open in a number of ways.

1. The solar plexus area is the only part of the body that is not covered by a bony structure. This is the center of your emotions. No creator would leave us without a way to keep this area clear; we can do it through the breath. Try this: lie down, relax as much as you can, and breathe from the diaphragm. Take in a breath and let everything out from the diaphragm. This will begin to allow energy to start to flow into that area; try to keep your mind only on your breathing. Even if you do this only five minutes a day, it will be beneficial; this type of breathing will also help tone the colon. At this time, you could also gently massage the colon from right to left. Breath is the first basic step to health.

2. Change your diet to a more natural one; stop eating the things that harm the body. Be kind to yourself. Feed yourself life-giving foods. Drink pure water. Educate yourself about nutrition. Nourishment is the second basic step to health.

3. Change your attitudes. Work with yourself. Be aware of how you feel about your own elimination processes. Love each thing about yourself. Don't put yourself down. Re-educate and reprogram yourself positively. In this physical world, your body is the house you live in; be comfortable in it. Accept it lovingly.

Clean the inner environment physically, emotionally, and mentally; no disease can flourish in a purified temple. In that type of environment, only the beauty of your own spirit and soul will grow.

Angela Bell is a licensed massage therapist who utilizes a holistic approach in her treatments. She also specializes in "Innerphasing," a reducing process that changes dietary habits.

Reprinted from Alternatives Magazine, *January 1978.*

Psychology of the Colon

by John Harvey Kellogg, M.D.

The colon is richly supplied with nerves and is highly sensitive to influence by all emotions pleasurable or the opposite. Studies have shown that unpleasant emotions of all sorts can stop peristalsis. Even very slight emotional excitement, as slight anxiety, annoyance, apprehension, or ill-temper may stop all movement of the intestines, as well as of the stomach, together with gastric secretions.

The colon, like the face, responds to every passing emotion. The intestines are perhaps more sensitive than are the muscles of the face to emotional excitement because they are more richly supplied with blood vessels and sympathetic nerves.

X-ray studies of animals have demonstrated the intimate association of the colon with the sympathetic nervous system and the profound effects of all forms of emotional excitement. When a dog was placed in strange surroundings, peristalsis within its colon ceased for several hours. When a cat, while under observation, had its tail pinched, peristalsis also ceased. The movements did not begin again until the cat was pacified and purring contentedly.

The depressing influence of fear is well established. The frightened colon cannot discharge its contents because the descending colon is in a spastic state. So long as the patient is fearful that his bowels will not move, they will not. The colon is in a state of stage fright. It is crippled; but all that is needed for a cure may be to get rid of apprehension and fear. In such a case, the most effective remedies will not move the bowels until the element of fear is removed. Confidence and faith can change the situation.

The angry colon shuts up like a clam and declares "no

thoroughfare here." Some persons are obstinately constipated because of a chronic state of ill will or anger.

Grief shuts up the outlet of the body's sewage system as tightly as does fear or anger. The worried colon neither secretes nor contracts. Both secretion and contraction are needed for efficient action—secretion for lubrication and contraction for transportation of the food residues to the exit. Loss of sleep, business worries, domestic trials, or harassment from any cause may render the colon dysfunctional.

In view of these facts, which might be multiplied at great length, it is evident that a right mental attitude as well as roughage and lubrication are essential for the successful treatment of a sluggish colon. With the laxative diet and various food accessories might be mingled the firm faith that the natural and biologic means employed will accomplish the desired outcome.

Such a faith will lead to regular visits to the toilet at the times when the bowels should move; that is, after each meal, on rising in the morning, and on going to bed at night. Do not wait for a "call," but invite a call by giving the colon a chance for evacuation and, by all means, avoid haste. A hurried visit to the toilet will not encourage normal colon activity. A slow colon must be given time, especially when by a change of diet and attention to colon hygiene it is just beginning to behave in something like a normal manner. By patient training, the sluggish bowel may after a time be trained to act with normal promptness and celerity.

From early infancy, the habit of prompt attention to the "call" for evacuation of the colon should be assiduously cultivated. Instead of doing this, the child is usually subjected to a process of housebreaking much like that to which house dogs are subjected. The result is the derangement of the natural order that empties the colon after each meal or three or four times a day. This establishes a crippled condition of the colon that permits but one evacuation a day, a form of constipation that is so universal among civilized people that it has come to be regarded as natural.

As soon as the child begins to run about, the mother begins to train him to restrain the movements of his bladder and bowels to suit convenience of time and place. A false sense of modesty also becomes a restraining influence that soon upsets the normal intestinal rhythm and lays the foundation for lifelong constipation and all the miseries associated with these conditions and the autointoxication to which they give rise.

Indeed, the majority of people and many physicians regard regularity as the essential element of colon health, and almost ignore the matter of frequency and thoroughness of evacuation. The late Sir Lauder Brunton, an eminent English internist, told of a lady who answered his inquiry about her colon function, "Perfectly regular, sir, perfectly regular." When further questioned, she disclosed the fact that although bowel movements were perfectly regular, they occurred only once in three weeks.

This article contains excerpts from Dr. John Harvey Kellogg's writing on colon health (1928). Dr. Kellogg founded the Battle Creek, Michigan, Sanitarium and the Kellogg's Breakfast Cereal Company.

Colon Therapy:
The Natural Way to Renewed Health

by Sheila Shea

We are all trained from early childhood to have very negative attitudes toward our organs of elimination. The colon and the anus are still taboo topics and people are not educated to treat their organs with care and respect.

Like millions of others who neglect their colons, I suffered through the years from chronic constipation, discomfort, and poor health. The constant muscle tensions were distorting my personality, and the accumulated toxins were poisoning my body, but all these problems were cleared up after I began the regular practice of watching my diet and cleansing my colon.

Actually, I was forced to confront my own digestive tract because I watched others in my family succumb to colon disorders. My father had cancer of the colon, my grandmother had severe intestinal problems, and my mother has been constipated much of her life. So, after I had undergone colonic therapy for a while, I decided to become a colon therapist. Now I have the continuing satisfaction of helping many people who suffer from distress of this vital organ.

A colonic is a gentle, warm-water washing of the colon or large intestine, combined with an external massage. At the foot of the massage table is a colon irrigation machine, which is simply a tank with tubing and a few levers and valves. One end of the tubing is put gently into the rectum.

Water flows into the colon, and when the client feels any pressure or discomfort, he or she asks for release. This process of filling and releasing is repeated until the colon is emptied. If desired, the contents of the colon may be viewed as they flow through a glass tube on their way to the drain.

A colonic usually lasts 45 minutes to an hour. While the water is leaving the colon, the irrigationist gives an abdominal massage in patterns to help eliminate gas, fecal matter, and mucous.

Most people are able to cleanse only about half of the colon by themselves via enemas. But, for a thorough cleansing of the entire colon—a high colonic—it is best to have the services of an experienced therapist.

My first introduction to colon irrigation came through Norman Walker's book *Raw Vegetable Juices* and the works of natural healer Arnold Ehret. Both authors believe that constipation is a basic cause of disease that can be remedied by dissolving the backlog of toxins and mucous. I began increasing my intake of citrus and vegetable juices to dissolve the mucous, but it wasn't until I was 31 that I had my first colon irrigation. I think I resisted getting one because I felt terribly ashamed of my chronic constipation. Also, from years of straining and resultant hemorrhoids, I had a very finnicky, sensitive anus, and I didn't like the thought of inserting anything into it.

However, a very close friend of mine had received a series of colonics and had encouraged me to do it, too. So we went to the Hippocrates Health Institute in Boston, and tried their diet of raw foods and vegetable juices for two weeks.

I still resisted the idea of a colonic, but my friend offered to go with me. As the institute's therapist began the colonic I burst into tears. My anal muscles were as tight as my jaw and neck muscles, and it was a truly emotional experience to try to loosen them. But I made it through the session and came back the next week for another—and they got easier and better as I became more accustomed to them.

Mine was an extreme case of dysfunction. In addition to my general physical problems, sex was often unpleasant for me.

The Colon Is a Neighbor

The colon lives in very close quarters with the kidneys, ovaries, bladder, and uterus or prostate gland. Roommates, if you will. In my case I had complaints ranging from vaginal infections and cystitis to herpes. Never once did I consider that any of these problems related to my colon.

I had been constipated for the first 26 years of life until I began taking enemas, a simple water cleansing of the colon using a standard two-quart bag. As I continued to cleanse my colon on a regular basis with colonics, fasting, raw juices, and more live foods, all of the symptoms of these infections disappeared and to this date have not returned.

You see, when the colon does not release its contents on a regular basis, the backlog of fecal matter putrefies. This putrefaction occurs through bacterial action. These bacteria multiply very rapidly and can pass through the walls of the colon to other organs. The bacteria begin the same process on these organs, which is to break down their proper function.

These bacteria create strong acids and gases that cause inflammation. They are ultimately released via the urethra or vaginal canal in the form of mucous or pus. The foods that these pathogenic or harmful bacteria thrive on are animal products, sugar, dairy, drugs, and chemicals.

When the slightest symptoms of these basic infections appear, the first thing to do is cleanse the colon and check your diet. If you have been indulging in any of the main offenders, lay off them. If your diet has been quite clean, then you are experiencing a cleansing of older material, remnants of that old diet of meat, dairy, sugar, salt, flour, and you know the rest.

I have also found that by adding a living primary yeast to my diet, I can minimize an infection to seven days and at the same time rejuvenate my immune system. I also suggest increasing the intake of green vegetables and fresh fruit. Harmful bacteria cannot thrive in an environment of greens and fruit.

All of the organs of the abdominal area are beautiful neighbors. It is a small but important community where cooperation, harmony, cleanliness, and comfort are of paramount value in maintaining and improving the quality of your health.

Focusing awareness and attention on the state of your colon is not only good hygiene and the prelude to natural healing—it is also an ancient form of yogic meditation. According to the yogic system, the body has seven centers of energy, or chakras. Each is an important center of psychic and physical energy, and all must function harmoniously and without impediment for the body to experience optimum health and well-being.

These centers are located at the anus, the sex organs, the solar plexus, the heart, the throat, the place between and above the eyes, and the top of the head. When there is distress or blockage in any of these centers, the entire balance of the body is thrown off. Yogis give sober attention, care, and meditation to each center. They feel its state from within— whether it is tense or relaxed, functioning smoothly or paralyzed with blockage. Yogic exercises are very useful for toning the abdomen; they can also be practiced during colonics.

People have asked me if I think it's unnatural to take so many enemas and colonics. With my history of chronic constipation, I have never known what is "natural." I find taking salt, sugar, chemicals, drugs, alcohol, highly refined foods, and not exercising on a regular basis "unnatural" for my body now. I think it's more "natural" in this society to be constantly ill, in pain, and constipated.

As a practicing colonic therapist, I've been astounded at all the fear, guilt, and shame people have built up. They're afraid they will "dirty" the table (that's what it's for), and they're embarrassed to talk about the process of elimination. The blackout in this culture about the whole lowest chakra or energy center, the anus, is almost total. Since the anus is the base of energy, balance, pleasure, power and security, to be constipated is literally to be "up tight."

Clients come to me for colon irrigation for many reasons: constipation, gas, sciatic pains, rheumatoid arthritis, cleansing to accompany diets, fasting, and pregnancy, cleansing before sex or an artistic performance, headaches (especially migraine), worms, after binges, in combination with diet change and weight loss, to combat poisoning from excess refined sugar, flour, and predigested animal protein—in short, for all problems caused by an overload of toxins in the body.

A few people come in tense, very hyper from the day's activities. Others talk compulsively on the table. Many try to hold back. In each case, the person has an inability to focus on his or her body and its physical functions. I tell each of them that colon irrigation is a meditation for the colon and that any kind of release is okay.

One potential client told me she was afraid to come in because of what I would see in the viewing tube. She wanted to get herself "clean" before she came in because she was afraid I would judge her and say her diet was bad and therefore she was bad. This is like cleaning house before your maid arrives, so she won't have a low opinion of your character.

Too many of my clients either hold in or push when they feel the pleasurable wave of release. Both actions constrict all the muscles in the lower pelvic bowel and prevent a cleansing. I call this reaction pleasure anxiety, and I teach people to let go of the closed-off sigmoid colon. Training people in the pleasure of releasing is part of a colonic therapist's job. I have achieved many breakthroughs using breathing, meditation, focus, massage, and water!

The factors that make cleansings more difficult are a prolapsed or fallen transverse colon; enlarged, impacted gas pockets; too much or too little muscle tone; a weak sigmoid colon; pushing or straining at the stool; and drugs that inhibit the colon.

Most people—including myself—have a prolapsed transverse colon.* The transverse has fallen like a hammock, usually to a point somewhere below the navel. The transverse then falls on other organs, such as the bladder or uterus, which in turn fall on the sigmoid colon and close it off.

Some causes of a prolapsed transverse colon are engorging the stomach with too much food, weak muscle tone from toxic diets and lack of exercise, poor posture, and impacted pockets.

There is a continuous series of one-to-two-inch pockets or saculations along the colon. These pockets enlarge when solids collect in them and are not eliminated. Decomposing meat and starches can even harden on the wall and cause a pocket to become impacted. When solids get stuck in the pockets, they putrefy or rot, creating more toxic wastes and gas, which expand the pockets further. I've had some marvelous results working out the contents of the pockets using various massage techniques. Abdominal massage is something you can do for yourself any time you want to loosen matter in the colon and stimulate peristalsis (alternating expansion and contraction of the entire digestive tube).

Most times gas is caused by improper food combinations, matter putrefying in pockets of the colon, mucous softening and being released from the colon wall, and inorganic toxic gases excreted by body cells.

The major improper combination is eating fruit or sugar with or after any starch, protein, or vegetable other than a green. When combined improperly, fruit, sugar, and alcohol ferment and cause gas, as well as expand gas that's already formed.

During a cleansing diet or a liquid fast, mucous is dislodged from the colon wall, often preceded by tremendous amounts of gas. Certain natural foods high in sulphur or chlorine, such as avocado or members of the cabbage family,

---

See page 11 for diagram.

release toxic gases by replacing them with natural ones. The gases are released more heavily when a person begins a natural food diet or a fast.

It is important to get gas out of the colon. As well as serving as a conduit for food wastes, the colon eliminates wastes from blood, lymph, liver, and nervous systems. When the colon is not being emptied regularly, these toxins are reabsorbed into the blood and nerves.

Drugs may also have an inhibiting effect on the colon. For example, antibiotics destroy the natural flora that live there and aid digestion. Certain chemicals, salts, and sugars in the diet have the same effect. Flora are not drawn from the colon wall with a water cleansing, but one candy bar wipes them out! Fresh fruit and vegetables, fermented foods, and unpasteurized yogurt and acidophilus continue to provide the colon with fresh flora.

A highly refined diet of salts, sugars, flours, fats, and dairy products causes mucous to harden on the walls of the colon. Although the body needs high-quality mucous in it at all times as a natural lubricant, "good" mucous has a liquid consistency and is derived from a diet of whole foods.

Good muscle tone in the abdomen is also essential for healthy elimination. Sometimes the abdominal muscles are overly tight from psychological tension or the wrong kind of abdominal exercises. Surgery can cause holding patterns in the muscles, also producing too much tension.

However, it is lack of muscle tone that is most common. When muscle tone is correct, involuntary contractions move solids, liquids, and gases rhythmically from one part of the body to the other.

For most people, gravity moves material through the colon. More input pushes what is already there a little bit farther down. Diet, exercise, and breathing—along with colonics or enemas—begin to stimulate peristalsis by breaking up large pockets of gas and impacted matter, loosening mucous, and toning abdominal muscles.

All in all, the benefits of high-colonic sessions are exercise of the rectal muscles, release of abdominal tension, the flushing out of accumulated toxins, and the relief of gas pains. Also, colon irrigation provides a chance for a person to take a break from his or her normal consciousness and focus on the true center of personal power—the colon. Restoring it to strong peristalsis, good tone, and harmonious functioning has a beneficial effect on your state of mind, your health, and your sex life.

Sheila Shea, D.D. is a Miami-based colon irrigationist who since 1970 has been devoted to self-healing and research on the colon.

Reprinted from Forum Magazine: The Journal of Human Relations, *Forum International, Ltd., 1978.*

CHAPTER 10

Quotes from America's Leading Experts on Colon Health

The Doctor
of the Future
Will give no medicine
But will interest his
Patient in the care of
The human frame, in diet,
And in the cause
And prevention of disease.

—Thomas A. Edison

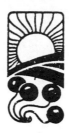

Quotes from Bernard Jensen, D.C., Ph.D.

- *It's often said that you are what you eat. I say that you are what you absorb.*

- *Insufficient numbers of bowel movements and too little fiber and bulk in the feces may often explain the existence of gall bladder disorders, heart problems, varicose veins, appendicitis, clotting in deep veins, hiatal hernia, diverticulosis, arthritis, and cancer of the colon.*

- *To try to take care of any symptom in the body without a good elimination is futile.*

- *I believe autointoxication is currently the number one source of the misery and decay we are witnessing in our society and culture today.*

- *The road to health is the one that begins with an understanding and commitment to cleanse and detoxify the body, to restore balance, peace, and harmony.*

- *The greatest healing power comes from within out.*

- *It takes an extreme measure of action and courage in order to get out of the bowel situation in which so many people find themselves. Knowing the ways of keeping the bowel healthy and in good shape is the best way I know to keep away from the grip of disease and sickness.*

- *The bowel-wise person is the one who is armed with good knowledge, practices discrimination in his eating habits, and walks the path of higher life. His days are blessed with health, vitality, optimism, and the fulfillment of life's goals. He is a blessing and source of inspiration to family associates. His cheerful disposition comes from having a vital, toxin-free body made possible by the efficient, regular cleansing action of a loved and well-cared-for bowel.*

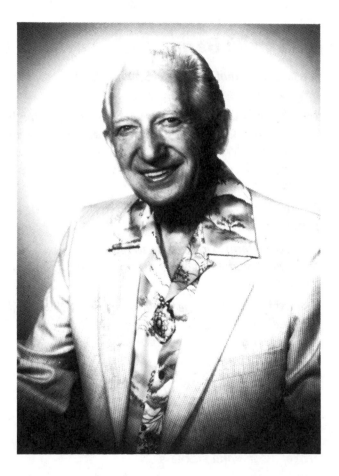

Bernard Jensen, D.C., Ph.D.

Quotes from Norman Walker, D.Sc.

- *Colon health emphasizes prevention rather than cure. It is the most important step in maintaining or regaining vital health.*

- *Colon irrigation along with other health programs have kept me ageless. No matter what—colon cleansings don't hurt you, they can only help you. If you think about it, they make sense.*

- *Most health enthusiasts don't realize that the colon is responsible for the assimilation of minerals and vitamins. Supplements at best are only partially absorbed with a clogged, encrusted, or heavily coated colon.*

- *Overweight is often the result of a backed-up system. Food stores rather than metabolizes.*

- *The hardened material that accumulates on the inside walls of the colon is like cement. It does not come down by itself, or with fasts, laxatives, enemas, or drugs, and it is at the root of many human problems.*

- *If the sewer system in your home is backed up, your entire home is affected. Should it be any different with your body?*

- *Don't just wait until your colon is completely blocked. Always think in terms of prevention. More than one million victims [of colon surgery] spent more than two billion dollars for surgery and convalescence, and that's only the beginning.*

- *The colon, just like the spine, is interrelated, interconnected, and interdependent with every other part of the body. Health in the colon often affects health in other areas of the body.*

- *Waste matter naturally collected in the colon and allowed to remain longer than necessary is by nature subject to fermentation and putrefaction, which is an area of toxicity that can be picked up by the bloodstream and settle in any part of your body.*

- *Colon irrigations help chiropractic adjustments keep, because of the decreased toxicity level. There is an interrelationship, one compliments the other.*

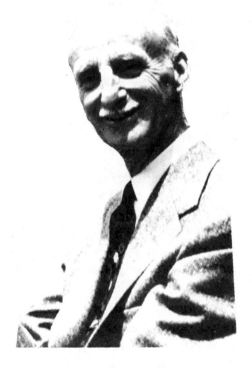

Norman W. Walker, D.Sc., as a centenarian.

Quotes by Norman W. Walker, D.Sc., are from his book *Colon Health: The Key to a Vibrant Life* (Norwalk Press, Prescott, Arizonia) and are used with his permission.

References & Suggested Reading

Abravanel, Elliot, M.D.
  Body Type Diet

Bieler, Henry, M.D.
  Food Is Your Best Medicine

Connolly, Pat
  The Candida Albicans Yeast Free Cookbook

Crook, William G., M.D.
  The Yeast Connection

Haas, Elson, M.D.
  Staying Healthy with the Seasons (Celestial Arts, 1981)

Harrower, Henry
  Practical Endocrinology

Jensen, Bernard, D.C., Ph.D.
  Tissue Cleansing Through Bowel Management (1981)
  Foods That Heal (Avery Publications, 1988)
  Love, Sex and Nutrition (Avery Publications, 1988)
  Vibrant Health From Your Kitchen
  Nature Has A Remedy
  Herbal Handbook

Kelley, William D., D.D.S.
  The Metabolic Types

Kellogg, John, M.D.
  Autointoxication or Intestinal Toxemia (Modern Medicine
      Publishing Company, 1922)

Kulvinskas, Viktoras
  Life in the 21st Century (Omangod Press, 1981)

Pottenger, Francis M., M.D.
  Symptoms of Visceral Disease

Rohe, Fred and Dr. William Kelley
  Metabolic Ecology: A Way to Win the Cancer War
      (Wedgestone Press, 1982)

Tilden, J.H., M.D.
Toxemia Explained
Appendicitis: The Etiology, Hygienic and Dietetic Treatment
(Health Research, 1976)

Trowbridge, John Parks, M.D. and Morton Walker, D.P.M.
The Yeast Syndrome

Truss, C. Orian, M.D.
The Missing Diagnosis

Valentine, Tom & Carole
Medicine's Missing Link

Walker, Norman, D.Sc.
Colon Health: The Key to a Vibrant Life (Norwalk Press)
Vibrant Health: The Possible Dream (Norwalk Press)
Raw Vegetable Juices (Norwalk Press, 1978)

Watson, George, Ph.D.
Nutrition and Your Mind, Personality Strength and Psychochemical Energy

Williams, Roger, Ph.D.
Biochemical Individuality:, Nutrition Against Disease

APPENDIX

Order Forms

Shipping and Handling

We ship both fourth class U.S. mail and surface U.P.S.

Shipping charges are shown on order forms.

For shipments to Alaska and Hawaii, double the continental U.S. shipping charge. Orders will be sent by air.

Foreign Orders

For surface shipments to Canada, double the continental U.S. shipping charge.

For overseas surface shipments, triple the shipping charge.

For air shipments overseas, add five (5) times the continental U.S. shipping charge.

Payment in U.S. Funds only.

Four- or Seven-Day
Colon Cleansing Program
Order Form

COLON HEALTH CENTER
P. O. Box 1013
Larkspur, CA 94939
(415) 924-6106

The Complete Four- or Seven-Day Colon Cleansing Program Kit Contains:

Bilax (8 tablets)	Dry Skin Brush
Castor Oil (16 oz.)	Flannel Cloth (for castor oil pack)
DDS-1 Acidophilus (100 caps.)	Pau D'Arco Tea (bulk pkg. 3 oz.)
Dr. Jensen's Broth (6 oz.)	Intestinal Cleanser (120 caplets)
KB-11 Tea (18 bags)	

	Quantity	Price	Total
Complete Four- or Seven-Day Colon Cleansing Program Kit	————	$65.00	————
Individual Items:			
Bilax (8 tablets)	————	1.00	————
Castor Oil (16 oz.)	————	12.00	————
DDS-1 Acidophilus (100 caps.)	————	16.00	————
Dr. Jensen's Broth (6 oz.)	————	5.00	————
Dry Skin Brush	————	5.00	————
Flannel Cloth	————	5.00	————
Pau D'Arco Tea (4 oz.)	————	8.00	————
Intestinal Cleanser (120 caplets)	————	8.00	————
KB-11 Tea (18 bags)	————	5.00	————

Total Order ————
California residents add 6% tax ————
Complete Kit postage & handling $7.00 ————
Postage & handling for individual items:
up to $50 add 10% of order price;
over $50 add 8% of order price ————
Amount Enclosed ————

Please complete the information form on the next page and send **both** pages.

Four- or Seven-Day
Colon Cleansing Program
Order Form

COLON HEALTH CENTER
P.O. Box 1013
Larkspur, CA 94939
(415) 924-6106

Continued from the previous page.
Please allow 2 weeks for delivery. Send check or money order payable to Colon Health Center. (No C.O.D.) Visa and MasterCard accepted. Prices subject to change. Please print clearly.

Name _____

Address _____

City, State, Zip _____

Telephone: Work ( ) _____ Home ( ) _____

VISA # └┴┴┴┴┴┴┴┴┴┴┴┴┴┴┴┴┘ Expir. Date _____

MC # └┴┴┴┴┴┴┴┴┴┴┴┴┴┴┴┘ Expir. Date _____

Signature _____

DDS-1 Acidophilus
Order Form

COLON HEALTH CENTER
P. O. Box 1013
Larkspur, CA 94939
(415) 924-6106

	Quantity	Price	Total
DDS-1 Acidophilus (100 capsules)	————	$16.00	————
Total Order			————
California residents add 6% tax			————
Postage & handling $1.50 per bottle			————
Amount Enclosed			————

Please allow 2 weeks for delivery. Send check or money order payable to Colon Health Center. (No C.O.D.) Visa and MasterCard accepted. Price subject to change. Please print clearly.

Name_____

Address_____

City, State, Zip_____

Telephone: Work (   ) _____ Home (   ) _____

VISA # └┘│││││││││││││││││┘ Expir. Date _____

MC # └┘││││││││││││││││││┘ Expir. Date _____

Signature _____

Eight-Week Candida Overgrowth Elimination Program Order Form

COLON HEALTH CENTER
P. O. Box 1013
Larkspur, CA 94939
(415) 924-6106

Eight-Week Candida Overgrowth Elimination Program Kit Contains:

Arizona Natural Garlic (1 bottle)   Kaprycidin-A (2 bottles)
Caprystatin (4 bottles)   Megavital (2 bottles)
Intestinal Cleanser (2 bottles)   Orithrush-D (1 bottle)
Co-Enzyme Q10 (2 bottles)   Pau D'Arco Tea (2 boxes)
DDS-1 Acidophilus (3 bottles)   Travacid X (2 bottles)

Product	Size	Quantity	Price	Total
Eight-Week Program Kit		_____	$326.00	_____

Individual Items:

Product	Size	Quantity	Price	Total
Ariz. Nat. Garlic	250 capsules	_____	12.00	_____
Caprystatin	90 tablets	_____	18.00	_____
Intestinal Cleanser	120 caplets	_____	8.00	_____
Co-Enzyme Q10	60 caps, 30 mg.	_____	21.00	_____
DDS-1 Acidophilus	100 capsules	_____	16.00	_____
Kaprycidin-A	90 capsules	_____	18.00	_____
Megavital	60 tablets	_____	19.00	_____
Orithrush-D	Liquid concen.	_____	14.00	_____
Pau D'Arco Tea	Bulk pkg. 3 oz.	_____	8.00	_____
Travacid X	100 tablets	_____	18.00	_____
The Yeast Syndrome	Book	_____	4.00	_____

Total Order   _____
California residents add 6% tax   _____
Complete Kit postage & handling $10.00   _____
Postage & handling for individual items: _____
    up to $50 add 10% of order price;
    over $50 add 8% of order price   _____
Amount Enclosed   _____

Please complete information form on the next page and send **both** pages.

Eight-Week Candida Overgrowth
Elimination Program
Order Form

COLON HEALTH CENTER
P. O. Box 1013
Larkspur, CA 94939
(415) 924-6106

Continued from the previous page.
Please allow 2 weeks for delivery. Send check or money order
payable to Colon Health Center. (No C.O.D.) Visa and MasterCard
accepted. Prices subject to change. Please print clearly.

Name _____

Address _____

City, State, Zip _____

Telephone: Work (   ) _____ Home (   ) _____

VISA # ⌊⌊⌊⌊⌊⌊⌊⌊⌊⌊⌊⌊⌊⌊⌊⌊⌊⌊⌊⌋ Expir. Date _____

MC # ⌊⌊⌊⌊⌊⌊⌊⌊⌊⌊⌊⌊⌊⌊⌊⌊⌊⌊⌊⌋ Expir. Date _____

Signature _____

Parasite Elimination Program
Order Form

COLON HEALTH CENTER
P. O. Box 1013
Larkspur, CA 94939
(415) 924-6106

If your weight is:	Quantity	Price	Total

Under 100 lbs. Complete 8-Week Kit _____ $ 134.00 _____
(2 bottles 6-N-1 Cleanser, 2 bottles Castor Oil Capsules, 2 bottles K-Min,
3 bottles DDS-1 Acidophilus, and 1 bottle Black Walnut Tincture)

101-175 lbs.   Complete 8-Week Kit _____ 162.00 _____
(3 bottles 6-N-1 Cleanser, 3 bottles Castor Oil Capsules, 2 bottles K-Min,
3 bottles DDS-1 Acidophilus, and 1 bottle Black Walnut Tincture)

Over 175 lbs.   Complete 8-Week Kit _____ 190.00 _____
(4 bottles 6-N-1 Cleanser, 4 bottles Castor Oil Capsules, 2 bottles K-Min,
3 bottles DDS-1 Acidophilus, and 1 bottle Black Walnut Tincture)

If your age is:
1–13 years   Complete 4-Week Kit _____ $ 80.00 _____
(Children's kit contains 1 bottle 6-N-1 Cleanser, 1 bottle Castor Oil Capsules,
1 bottle K-Min, 2 bottles DDS-1 Acidophilus, and 1 bottle Black Walnut
Tincture)

Individual Items:
6-N-1 Intestinal Cleanser (250 caps.) _____ $ 16.00 _____
Castor Oil (180 capsules) _____ 12.00 _____
K-Min (180 capsules) _____ 10.00 _____
Black Walnut Tincture (4 oz.) _____ 10.00 _____
DDS-1 Acidophilus (100 capsules) _____ 16.00 _____

> **Total Order**
> California residents add 6% tax _____
> Complete Kit postage & handling $10.00 _____
> Postage & handling for individual items: _____
>   up to $50 add 10% of order price;
>   over $50 add 8% of order price _____
> **Amount Enclosed** _____

Please complete information form on the next page and send
both pages.

Parasite Elimination Program
Order Form

COLON HEALTH CENTER
P. O. Box 1013
Larkspur, CA 94939
(415) 924-6106

Continued from the previous page.
Please allow 2 weeks for delivery. Send check or money order payable to Colon Health Center. (No C.O.D.) Visa and MasterCard accepted. Prices subject to change. Please print clearly.

Name_____

Address_____

City, State, Zip_____

Telephone: Work (   ) _____ Home (   ) _____

VISA # |__|__|__|__|__|__|__|__|__|__|__|__|__|__|__|__| Expir. Date _____

MC # |__|__|__|__|__|__|__|__|__|__|__|__|__|__|__|__| Expir. Date _____

Signature _____

HEALING WITHIN:
The Complete Colon Health Guide
Book Order Form

COLON HEALTH CENTER
P. O. Box 1013
Larkspur, CA 94939
(415) 924-6106

	Quantity	Price	Total
HEALING WITHIN: *The Complete Colon Health Guide*	_____	$8.95	_____
Total Order			_____
California residents add 6% tax			_____
Postage & handling $1.00 per book			_____
Amount Enclosed			_____

Please allow 2 weeks for delivery. Send check or money order payable to Colon Health Center. (No C.O.D.) Visa and MasterCard accepted. Price subject to change. Please print clearly.

Name _____

Address _____

City, State, Zip _____

Telephone: Work ( ) _____ Home ( ) _____

VISA # |_|_|_|_|_|_|_|_|_|_|_|_|_|_|_|_|_|_| Expir. Date _____

MC # |_|_|_|_|_|_|_|_|_|_|_|_|_|_|_|_|_|_| Expir. Date _____

Signature _____

WHOLESALE INQUIRIES WELCOMED

Let us not criticize adversely or condemn matters regarding which we are not fully informed. There are always two sides to every question.

Who can tell which is right and which is wrong?

Experience alone proves that no one man has all the answers.

—Norman W. Walker, D. Sc., 1955

This page is left blank for your notes